Praise WELLNESS WISDOM

"*Wellness Wisdom* lifted my energy immediately . . . This book contains a powerful blueprint for what wellness looks and feels like."

~Christiane Northrup, M.D.
Author of *Women's Bodies, Women's Wisdom, Mother-Daughter Wisdom, The Wisdom of Menopause,* and *The Secret Pleasures of Menopause*

"Susan Tate is a joyful, enthusiastic, cosmic cheerleader for life, health, and consciousness. She has managed the almost impossible task of making transformational reading fun and inviting. *Wellness Wisdom* is a beautiful synthesis of timeless teachings for wellness on all levels—body, mind, heart, and soul. I trust you'll enjoy the tasty medicine it offers ..."

~Marc David
Nutritional Psychologist and author of *Nourishing Wisdom* and *The Slow Down Diet: Eating for Pleasure, Energy, & Weight Loss*

"Susan Tate weaves stories, humor, wisdom, and science in this easily accessible guide to wellness. I love that it is organized into 31 delicious bites of wellness wisdom. What a perfect way to integrate wellness into a busy lifestyle! This second edition takes the reader from inspiration to action—right into joyful wellness. My favorite way to use this book is to read one section each day—and then to continue re-reading month after month in order to spiral deeper and deeper into wellness."

~Deborah Kern, Ph.D.
Author of *Everyday Wellness for Women* and co-author of *Create the Body Your Soul Desires*

Wellness Wisdom

Also by Susan Tate
(Written under her former name, Susan Tate Firkaly)

Into the Mouths of Babes: A Natural Foods Nutrition and Feeding Guide for Infants and Toddlers

AIDS & HIV Education: Effective Teaching Strategies

Working Together to Prevent Sexual Assault (with Mark S. Benn, Psy.D.)

Wellness Wisdom

◆

31 Ways
to
Nourish Your
Mind, Body, & Spirit

Susan Tate

iUniverse, Inc.
New York   Bloomington

Wellness Wisdom
31 Ways to Nourish Your Mind, Body, & Spirit

Note to the reader: This book is meant to support and guide you as you make choices to enhance your well-being. The information in this book has been prepared thoughtfully and carefully. It is not intended to be prescriptive or diagnostic, nor is it a substitute for medical advice or treatment. Contact a qualified healthcare professional if you need medical assistance.

Edited by Liane Thomas
Cover design by Crista Goddard
Cover photo © 2006, Natalia Bratslavsky
Photo by Donna Lowe

iUniverse books may be ordered through booksellers or by contacting:

iUniverse
1663 Liberty Drive
Bloomington, IN 47403
www.iuniverse.com
1-800-Authors (1-800-288-4677)

Because of the dynamic nature of the Internet, any Web addresses or links contained in this book may have changed since publication and may no longer be valid. The views expressed in this work are solely those of the author and do not necessarily reflect the views of the publisher, and the publisher hereby disclaims any responsibility for them.

ISBN: 978-1-4502-7309-1 (sc)
ISBN: 978-1-4502-7310-7 (ebk)

Library of Congress Control Number: 2010918111

Printed in the United States of America

iUniverse rev. date: 1/19/2011

To a vision of a peaceful planet

through

individual, community, and global wellness.

No one can give you wisdom.
You must discover it for yourself,
on the journey through life,
which no one can take for you.

~Sun Bear

Contents

In Gratitude xiii

Introduction to the Second Edition xvii

Introduction to the First Edition xxi

Wellness Bill of Rights xxiii

CHAPTER 1 Intend to Be Well 1

CHAPTER 2 Listen to Your Body 8

CHAPTER 3 Actively Participate in Your Health 10

CHAPTER 4 Observe How You Talk to Your Body 14

CHAPTER 5 Nourish the Body/Mind 17

CHAPTER 6 Gently Seek Balance and Joy 26

CHAPTER 7 Honor the Body/Mind Temple 32

CHAPTER 8 Know God 34

CHAPTER 9 Pray and Meditate 37

CHAPTER 10 Live! 42

CHAPTER 11 Create a Monthly Focus 47

CHAPTER 12 Spend Money with Joy and Wisdom 51

CHAPTER 13 Cultivate Forgiveness 57

CHAPTER 14 Practice Peace 61

CHAPTER 15 Discover the Joys of Movement 67

CHAPTER 16 Revel in Relaxation 71

CHAPTER 17 Reframe Worrying 77

CHAPTER 18 Letting Go 81

CHAPTER 19 Laugh Often 84

CHAPTER 20 Embrace Intimacy 86

CHAPTER 21 Love Radically 89

CHAPTER 22   Enjoy Conscious Sexuality 94

CHAPTER 23   Honor Orgasms 99

CHAPTER 24   Be a Good Receiver 102

CHAPTER 25   Eliminate Clutter 104

CHAPTER 26   Be a Lifelong Learner .109

CHAPTER 27   Take a Well Day 111

CHAPTER 28   Practice Mindfulness .113

CHAPTER 29   Live in the Present Moment 115

CHAPTER 30   Don't Complain 117

CHAPTER 31   Magnify Gratitude 120

Closing Thoughts 123

Affirmations for Wellness 125

Wellness Action Plan 126

Bibliography 128

Reflection Pages 132

About the Author 142

In Gratitude

It is with an abundance of gratitude that I sit to write these pages to acknowledge those who contributed to this book. My own wellness wisdom didn't come to me in isolation. Life experiences with family, friends, colleagues, teachers, clients, students, and people I've met only briefly have contributed to the book you now hold in your hands. I am grateful to all who have enhanced my wellness wisdom.

Prayers and blessings flow to . . .

Helen and Ray Tate, my late parents, for the gift of life and for your profound love.

My siblings: Jack Tate, Patrick Tate, Beth Evers, and the late Cynthia Lamb—thank you for the gift of learning from you as I continue to grow in recognizing both our differences and our similarities.

Karen King, my goddess friend in St. Catharines, Ontario, for constantly holding a space for me to remember who I really am.

Phyllis Fontana, for sharing your wisdom and pragmatic beliefs that have been instrumental in keeping me grounded and balanced.

Ms. Lowe, thank you, Donna, for always being there to add your impish laughter, incredible compassion, and constant support of my writing (and other) endeavors coast-to-coast and decade-to-decade.

Fran Howard, for mirroring the best of who we are, for teaching me about the language of non-violent communication, for sharing your vast wisdom, and for listening without judging.

Barbara Black, for your radiant, courageous presence in my life and on this planet.

Ron and Cheryl Lewis, for your faithful friendship and love throughout the decades of learning life's lessons in wellness, loving, and living.

Liane Thomas, my copyeditor (all one word) queen. Your expertise, humor, support, gentle encouragement, and knack for deleting (and adding) commas are reflected in the quality of this book.

Crista Goddard, for your talented graphic design skills in our co-creation of the book cover. Your generous heart and shining light added much to this work.

Cindy Janechild, for always believing in me, for your healing magic, and for giving it to me straight.

Howard Bloom, for your faithful friendship and support; and for your constant reminder that the part of Susan Tate is being perfectly played by Susan Tate.

Debbie Rosas and Carlos AyaRosas, the co-creators of The Nia Technique, Inc. Your magnificent wisdom and creation of Nia has had a profound effect on my mind, body, spirit, and emotions.

My first Nia teacher, Chris Friedman, for holding a space and belief in my ability to teach Nia.

The Nia Seattle community of teachers and students, I am blessed to dance through this part of life with you.

My clients, for the honor of witnessing your wellness journeys and for what you teach me in the process.

The special friends and family members who provided their edits and comments for the final manuscript: Beth Evers, Cindy Janechild, Fran Howard, Karen King, Donna Lowe, Lee Ann Romberger, and Sarah Sheehan.

Lynn Hughes, for your Web design genius and sharing of your brilliant mind and heart.

Dr. Christiane Northrup, Marc David, Debbie Rosas, Dr. Deborah Kern, and Dr. Karen Wolfe for taking the time to read this manuscript and for providing such supportive endorsements.

My Team Northrup colleagues, whose vision of a healthier world inspires and supports the wellness of people across the globe.

My sangha sisters: Anita Faunlander, Christina Halas, Leslie Haines, Roberta Nelson, Denise Merrill, Kara Pomeroy, Katie Riss, and Jody Walmsley for years of prayer support and constant flow of wisdom.

Rev. Dr. Kathianne Lewis and the Center for Spiritual Living in Seattle for the teachings that have expanded my heart and faith; for teaching me to love who I am right now, for the idea of prosperity consciousness, and for helping me to broaden my ever-deepening faith in God.

My colleagues who worked with me through the years at the University of Virginia, for supplying me with such a supportive and safe environment to thrive and deepen my wellness wisdom.

The many wise women and men referenced in this book for having such an impact on my beliefs, thoughts, and attitudes.

My grandchildren, Abu and Aurora—the next generation of wise souls. Thank you for your wit, laughter, and love … and to the mother of these precious ones, Peggy Farley, for your wondrous and expansive mothering heart.

My step-grandchildren: Jack, Mattie Ree, Ruby, Johanna, and George. Thank you for the reminder that love continues in the most precious of ways.

My first husband, Michael Firkaly. From high school sweethearts to marriage partners, from parents to lifelong friends … thank you for all the love, for our children, and for the life experiences that expanded my wisdom at a profound soul level.

John Lockney, my second (and now former) husband, for providing me with rich opportunities to grow through love, laughter, tears, and learning. My wellness wisdom is deeply connected to our life experiences both together and apart.

Nalani Williams, for loving my son, for being all you are, and for being in my life.

Patrick Peter Polascek, the awesome Austrian man who makes my daughter laugh and reflects the presence of love in her daily life.

Zack Orion and Molly Firkaly, the most spectacular children I could have ever wished for—oh what you two have taught me! Thank you for the gift of watching you grow and flourish as the creative, compassionate, and wise individuals that you are.

The Wondrous Wise One of All, thank you, God, for my amazing life and for the precious opportunity to share this wisdom with others.

Introduction to the Second Edition

Well. Well. Well. Is that how you want to feel? Then I've written this book for you so you can experience more joy and wholeness in your every day life.

My first edition of *Wellness Wisdom: 31 Ways to Nourish Your Mind, Body, & Spirit* offered bite-sized morsels packed with information and inspiration to nourish your wellness journey. Three years later, this expanded edition is intended to move you from inspiration to action so you may transition from the "appetizer" to the "main course".

In 2009, as the heat of the U.S. healthcare reform debates melted into and through the media, I observed it with a sense of sad fascination. As a health and wellness educator for many decades, I watched as the focus of these debates centered on disease, fear, and illness care—rather than on strategies for promoting health and preventing illness.

But healthcare reform can only do so much, and most of it happens after the fact. In these times, more than ever, I want to share ways to prevent chronic degenerative disease and support your own plan of optimal wellness, even if you deal with a life-threatening condition or chronic illness. I am passionate about inspiring and empowering people to take responsibility for nourishing their mind, body, and spirit. This second edition is my way of presenting a powerful, sustainable, and cost-effective plan for "Wellness Care Reform."

In this edition, you'll find a combination of the latest science-based and mind/body healing strategies. These chapters now include practical lists to guide you toward deepening your wellness practice or meditations to nourish you. And right before the first chapter, I offer a Wellness Bill of Rights to support you in creating your own responsible healthcare reform.

As you'll read in the Introduction to the first edition of *Wellness Wisdom*, I learned earlier in life "how to be sick well." When I was a young mother, I was highly skilled at juggling career and home, missing meals and sleep, and working extra hours to help make ends meet. I was really great at taking care of everyone else around me, and the word "self-care" wasn't in my vocabulary. It seemed I was always getting sick. How ironic, since I was a high school health education teacher at the time.

I spent 17 years teaching health education to 16-year-olds—and left high school teaching when I had a 16-year-old of my own! During those years, I taught my students a variety of health topics including: human sexuality, mental health, nutrition, substance abuse, disordered eating, thanatology (the study of death and dying), stress management, decision-making, and effective communication. I was passionate about educating and empowering these teens to view their lives and bodies as precious.

In 1983 I experienced a surgical accident that required life-saving surgery and a massive blood transfusion. It was in the early days of the AIDS epidemic and fortunately the blood I received was virus-free; but the experience was a major turning point in my life.

I was unable to work for several months (I was teaching at Charlottesville High School in Virginia at the time), my immune system was shot, I experienced episodes of depression, and wore my comforting purple chenille bathrobe around the house for quite some time. It was the perfect attire for my personal pity party.

Over time, and with much support, I eventually chose to focus on wellness rather than illness—but it wasn't always an easy choice. During those unexpected months at home, I eventually created time (and found energy) to organize the research I had been gathering on the topic of infant nutrition. A year later, my first book, *Into the Mouths of Babes*, was published.

When I returned to the classroom, I added AIDS education to my course syllabus (HIV/AIDS wasn't yet a part of the vernacular), so my high school students would have information, skills, and support to make safer decisions. This led to my second book, *AIDS Education: Effective Teaching Strategies*. After the second edition of this book was published, I was propelled out of high school teaching into the world of college health when I was asked to be a consultant for the American College Health Association. Through a cooperative grant with the Centers for Disease Control (CDC), I had the opportunity to travel across the country to provide HIV/AIDS education training for college health professionals. (By the way, I love that the CDC has added the word "Prevention" to its name, as we know it today as the Centers for Disease Control and Prevention.) This ultimately landed me a position at the University of Virginia as the director of health promotion and assistant professor in the School of Medicine. During my tenure there, I proposed, developed, and taught the first-ever sexuality class at this university. It was during this time that I wrote my third book, *Working Together to Prevent Sexual Assault.*

In the transition from secondary education to the world of college health, another major life event occurred that had a profound effect on my personal and professional life —I discovered The Nia Technique. This powerful lifestyle practice that combines martial arts, dance arts, and healing arts was instrumental in literally keeping me upright during some pretty intense years of grief and loss. As a certified black belt Nia instructor, I have discovered that joyful movement is essential to the nourishment of the mind, body, and spirit. You can read more about Nia in Chapter 15.

In 2000, I followed my soul's longing to move to the Pacific Northwest. In August of that year I created Washington Wellness Associates and dwell in gratitude for my many opportunities to show how wellness is communicable. I get a kick out of sharing my wellness wisdom through presentations, workshops, books, Nia, and consulting.

This is how my wellness care reform unfolded. Through the life events laced in the above chronology, I slowly realized the importance of taking care of myself before trying to "save the world." The accidents and illnesses faded into the past and have been replaced with a conscious intent to be well. Along with this intention is my desire for others to be well too.

I trust this second edition will provide a concrete guide to assist you in transforming your thoughts and feelings into powerful action steps for supporting your wellness vision. Some of you may have experienced similar stages in life where illness was your focal point. If you are truly inspired to shift your focus off the illness or condition that may describe symptoms you have—symptoms that neither describe you nor who you are—then this second (main course) edition will nourish and guide you. If you already practice amplifying your wellness, this book will be a healthy dessert to add delight to your mind, body, and spirit.

You'll find a Wellness Action Plan and Reflection Pages in the back of this revised edition. You may want to ask a trusted friend (or gather a small group together) to join you in this process. Take your time, seek pleasure, and always add your own intuition and wisdom as you nourish your mind, body, and spirit.

I am sending my best to you as you journey deeper into wholeness. Be well.

Introduction to the First Edition

I spent more than half of my life learning how to "be sick well." Now I treasure the joys of being well. During my years as a young mother, I subconsciously believed that being sick was the only way I could get a rest and have someone take care of *me* for a while. It took many years for me to discover that *I* was the best person to take care of me. I now know that if I am well, I have much more to give to my family, friends, profession, and community. You may find the same to be true for you.

Wellness Wisdom: 31 Ways to Nourish Your Mind, Body, & Spirit, is intended to fill you with knowledge, skills, and support that will ultimately enhance all aspects of your wellness journey. Wellness is a choice and a lifetime process, not a final destination. You will always have the opportunity to choose where you want to go, what you want to bring, and what you want to leave behind as you continue on your own unique path.

Flight attendants have a great way of reminding us how important it is to take care of ourselves first. When giving instructions for the use of oxygen masks, they say, "If you are traveling with small children, or someone who needs assistance, put *your* mask on first before helping others." Once I realized it was important and even acceptable to take care of *me*, I stopped getting sick all the time. I am now making better choices on my own precious path of wellness.

I invite you to intuitively decide how to read this book. You may choose to read the entire book at once or you may prefer to linger on one of the 31 chapters each day for a month, taking in details of a particular topic. I trust you will discover, as you read each chapter, I make no attempt to use blame, shame, or guilt as you make changes in your life. Trust yourself to take what works for you and put aside any idea that might not feel comfortable for your lifestyle or beliefs. Be observant and make your choices with love.

As you create or re-create your own personal philosophy of wellness, listen to your body's wisdom and let it be your guide. The more frequently you tune in, the more easily you can listen to its loving whispers and harness the vitality that is uniquely yours. Allow your new ways of nourishing your mind, body, and spirit to fill you up and sustain you.

It is a privilege and an honor to share *Wellness Wisdom* with you. Thank you for taking the time to add these ideas to your own wisdom, culture, and beliefs. I wish you much joy as you journey.

Wellness Bill of Rights

I have the right to feel healthy, happy, and whole.

I have the right to set the intention to be as well as I can be, even if I have a chronic or life-threatening illness.

I have the right to choose vibrant, wholesome foods that nourish my mind, body, and spirit.

I have the right to dedicate several hours a week to exercise (movement) that I love.

I have the right to leave work or home to take a pleasurable walk every day of the week.

I have the right to refrain from putting the word "my" in front of any diagnosis of illness I may have received.

I have the right to choose thoughts that transform worry into mindful peace.

I have the right to forgive.

I have the right to take the stairs more often and count my blessings on each step.

I have the right to dance like no one is watching.

I have the right to park farther away from my destination.

I have the right to meditate and pray.

I have the right to give and receive love freely.

I have the right to support a more nourishing selection and supply of foods for children across the globe.

I have the right to support the provision of healthy food offered through government food subsidies for low-income people.

I have the right to support the educational and other wellness needs of women and girls worldwide so that centuries of abuse can end.

I have the right to play the leading role in decision-making for all of my health care needs.

I have the right to take advantage of screenings for the early detection of illness.

I have the right to choose high-quality supplements that nourish my body at a cellular level.

I have the right to die healthy after many decades of wondrous living.

I have the right to die with dignity in the place where I choose.

I have the right to create a living will.

I have the right to designate a durable power of attorney for health care to make my decisions if I become incapacitated.

I have the right to read books (like this one!) that uplift my spirit and support my well-being.

1

Intend to Be Well

○ ○

Intention is like an arrow flying toward a target.

—*Sonia Choquette*

One of the most powerful steps you can take to enhance your wellness is to simply create the intention to do so. Wellness is about choice. Wellness is the part of our well-being that describes what we have, rather than something we're lacking. When we're sick it's easy to proclaim to anyone who will listen, "I am so sick!" When we are well, we rarely walk around saying, "Oh, I am so well!" But the mind would love to hear this message more often. You might even make wellness communicable simply by talking about it!

Wellness is an active process, a choice, and a way of life. When we intend to be well, we make proactive choices that enhance our lives so that we feel more successful in all areas of our existence. That's wellness—and you want more of it or you wouldn't be reading this book.

When we focus on wellness, our wellness expands. In contrast, focusing on illness usually keeps us ill. You can choose to keep focusing on illness or you can begin to observe your thoughts, make a choice to change them, and create more episodes of spontaneous wellness in your life. You can enhance your level of wellness even if you have a chronic or serious illness. Setting the intention or stating a goal engages your mind to begin creating thoughts, feelings, ideas, and images of being and staying well. Affirming that you are already enjoying an abundance of wellness engages your subconscious to provide the spark that can light the flame of wellness within you. It also raises your energetic vibration so you can attract more of the same.

In setting intentions, you will want to involve your thoughts, words, and feelings, and then add a plan of action to your vision. Simply thinking about wellness more than sickness will get you moving in the right direction and writing down your intention is powerful. However, if you stopped there and sat in your living room waiting for wellness to walk in the door, you might be waiting for a while. It is important for your intention (thought) and word to be combined with feeling and then to be followed up with action. Identifying and drawing in the feeling that surrounds what you want is a very important step in this process.

We have over 60,000 thoughts a day. How many of your thoughts today are proclaiming your wellness? Do you spend time thinking or talking about what you *want* in your life or about what you *don't want*? Your answer to that question is important because what you think about all the time is what you will experience. Another way to say that is: What you think about expands. Think back over this past week and recall where you put your attention as it related to the concepts of wellness or illness. Did you spend time thinking about what part of your body didn't work right or were you focusing on moving toward a higher level of wellness? Did your conversations include more talk of aches and pains, or joy and ease? Sometimes it seems that we're all in a contest to see whose story holds the most pain or sickness. The winner really is *not* the one who feels worse than you! Giving wellness your attention will strengthen your intention to feel better than you do right now.

I have noticed I often avoid colds or minimize the symptoms of a cold by honoring my body's need for rest and by not over-scheduling myself. But I wasn't always this healthy. My old medical records are quite thick and several years ago I looked over them with amazement. I found page after page of notes describing conditions I haven't even thought of in the last 20 years. Back in 1984, one doctor actually wrote in my chart, "She is overburdening herself which leaves her no time for herself and the only way she gets taken care of is by getting sick." Ouch! My wellness path took a startling new direction after I realized that I seemed to be having accidents or illnesses in order for people to take care of me. None of this was at all conscious. Up until that time, I really didn't know how to take care of myself because I was too busy taking care of everyone around me. This focus of taking care of others while ignoring my own needs was in my DNA (and I swear it's in estrogen) so I spent a lot of time putting others first. Does this story sound familiar?

This awareness shifted my life considerably. I began to observe my thoughts, feelings, and actions surrounding illness. This shift continued when I became acutely aware of the thoughts I attached to my first sniffle or sneeze. I had developed quite a talent for planning ahead to feel miserable—I could even envision how many days I would be off work. That was after the first sneeze! I now make the choice to "think well" rather than to "think sick." Instead of believing, "Oh, I'm going to be so sick!" I declare, "I am well, I am well, I am well!" On rare occasions I might still find myself dealing with a minor cold, but it passes quickly and I don't pay much attention to it. Instead I pay more attention to myself and ask, "What can I do to take care of myself today?" I have also learned not to criticize myself when I am sick, thinking that I "should" have been able to avoid the illness.

Sometimes, despite our best intentions, we just get sick. When that happens, pamper yourself and let others pamper you too, if that's what you like. Sometimes we may just need the time to slow down and stay under the covers. And sometimes life deals us a chronic or life-threatening illness that we didn't ask for. In those cases, we can still focus on what *is* working in our body and create ways to be as well as we can be, despite our illness.

If you want to feel better and you don't feel well now, allow yourself to daydream to remember how it felt when you were in better health. Act as if you feel well and keep focused on the feeling that is behind your intention. The result will be magical.

You can choose to put your attention toward being well and to treat your body the best you can all the time, not just when you are sick. You can also observe, rather than judge, your patterns and choose to create new ones that may better serve your well-being.

One way to create new patterns is to take stock of what you do to fill yourself up each day. Many years ago as a graduate student in a stress management class, I was introduced to the concept of a *wellness bucket*. We actually took crayons and paper and drew our own personal bucket. Inside the bucket we wrote the things that we do to keep ourselves filled up, nourished, energized, and healthy. In other words, we wrote down what we did to keep our level of wellness high and our wellness bucket full. Then we used our artistic talents to depict the life stressors that poked holes in our bucket or caused our wellness to spill out. I remember my bucket was leaking in several places. It was such a strong visual that I still remember it years later.

The idea behind this concept is to be sure we are always adding to our bucket, always filling it up again. Daily life, by its nature, depletes our wellness supply. Some big life events completely dry up the inside of the bucket and poignant, painful passages seem to create cracks that take much time to heal. Fortunately, life also gives us the opportunity to overflow with health, happiness, and joyful wellness. Constantly replenishing your bucket is the goal. Think of it as your personal wellness savings bank—you want to keep making deposits. You can even create your own (Wellness) Bucket list, inspired by the Jack Nicholson and Morgan Freeman film, *The Bucket List*. Instead of making a list of things you might want to do before you "kick the bucket," this list is about your own personal bucket of wellness—things that fill up your bucket and things that poke holes in it *now*.

So, if you like, pull out some crayons and paper and create a drawing of your own wellness bucket. What would you place inside? You may include things like meditation, walking, Nia, yoga, painting, reading, nourishing foods, listening to music, getting enough sleep, making love, praying, laughing, connecting with family, Pilates, hiking, camping, volunteering, bicycling, taking supplements, curling up with your pet, enjoying a bubble bath, playing or watching your favorite sport, talking with a friend, going out to lunch . . . the wellness list is endless.

Then gently observe and put on paper the things that make your bucket leak. You can make things pour out the top, leak out the sides or pierce through the bottom. It's your bucket! Note things that deplete your wellness stores. They may include illness, work stress, the death of someone dear, family stress, money concerns, too many responsibilities, relationship wounds, traffic, long commutes, critical self-talk, too much e-mail, sugary or processed foods . . . and yes, this list is endless too. To benefit most from this activity, take a moment to commit to choosing something you will do every day to keep your bucket filled or replenished.

Or if you aren't up for an art activity, you may want to take the time now to create an intention statement or affirmation for your overall wellness and wholeness. You can get some good ideas in the list of wellness affirmations at the end of this book. Write your intention and put it on your refrigerator or bathroom mirror for a daily reminder. Underneath your statement, write down two actions you can take to make this intention a reality. Be sure to make your statement in the present rather than in the future and focus on what you will *do* rather than *not do*. One good example is, "I am joyfully focusing on my wellness by choosing nourishing foods." That works better than "I will be healthier because I will not eat as many cookies." The latter statement will put the responsibility of your wellness out there, somewhere in the future. And if you focus on NOT eating cookies, your mind will hungrily remember the word *cookies* and ignore the word *not*! We all know what happens when someone tells us *not* to think of the pink dancing elephant in the living room; see? The next step is to spend at least 17 seconds drawing the *feeling* to you that would result once your intention has unfolded. I have been learning that this *feeling* step is crucial to creating meaningful changes in my life. Try it!

I also encourage you to remove anything on your fridge or computer that discourages you, shames you, or sends negative messages that don't really motivate you. Be gentle and loving with yourself as you continue with this process. You have a lot of choices on your wellness journey. Enjoy them!

You'll find a Wellness Action Plan worksheet in the back of this book. When you are ready to set your goals and create a plan to enhance your level of wellness, you will enjoy taking time to create your customized plan. The concepts provided in this book can be added to your own wisdom and intuition so you can create the perfect plan. You may want to read the Wellness Bill of Rights at the beginning of this book before you complete your action plan.

You will also find Reflection Pages in the back of this book. You are invited to note your thoughts, feelings, and plans as you move from chapter to chapter. You can even play with drawing your wellness bucket on one of these pages if you like. My wish is that you use this book to nourish YOU as you personalize, process, and envision your next best steps into deeper wellness.

After you set the *in*tention, then put your *at*tention to it. Add the sensation of the feeling and you'll find this to be a simple yet powerful concept. An old proverb states, "If you plant turnips you will not harvest grapes." What seeds of wellness are you planting? What would you like to harvest?

Five Suggestions to Guide You in Creating Your Intention

1. Take a few moments to reflect on the last several days and bring to mind how you spoke or thought about your health. (Example: "Oh, I am so tired today." Or "My arthritis is acting up again," or, "I feel good but I'd like to feel even better!"

2. How do you want to feel? Close your eyes and take 17 seconds to dream, visualize, and imagine how you would feel if you were stronger, healthier, had less pain, or enjoyed a higher level of wellness than you are experiencing right now.

3. Create an intention statement, in the present tense, that will direct your attention toward expanding you level of wellness. (See the Affirmations for Wellness on page 125 for ideas to guide you. You may also want to take a look at the Wellness Action Plan and answer the first several questions.

4. Create your Wellness Bucket so you can identify what depletes you and what fills you.

5. Write three action steps you can take within the next few days that will lead you closer to your intention. Write them on a calendar or place them in a prominent spot.

2

Listen to Your Body

○ ○

There is vitality, a life force, an energy, a quickening, that is translated through you into action, and because there is only one of you in all time, this expression is unique. And if you block it, it will never exist through any other medium and will be lost.

—*Martha Graham*

How many times have you ended up with a horrible cold or the flu after pushing yourself through days, weeks, or months without really nurturing your body? Your body may have been quietly sending you messages during that time to get more rest, drink more water, eat nourishing foods, or take time to re-energize. Pausing frequently to listen to your body might be easier than waiting until illness forces you to slow down.

Do you have days when you bump into furniture, drop things, forget things, and feel unusually disorganized? These are often the kinds of messages your body sends to help you get back into the present moment and pay more attention to the *now*. It seems like it would be easy to take time to listen to your body, yet this is a challenging task to do while flying through the day as if you were on a non-stop flight. You *can* make the nourishing choice to slow down, listen, and even re-fuel now and then.

Our body's wisdom is always available to us. If we tune in, we can more easily listen to its loving whispers, accessing a vitality that is uniquely ours. Enjoy your whispering wisdom.

Here is a wonderful body scan exercise for you to enjoy. I invite you to read this next paragraph through, then close your eyes and begin your body scan.

Body Scan

Stand for a moment with your eyes closed and your bare feet resting comfortably beneath your hips. Take a few deep breaths, and settle your weight evenly over both feet. Draw an imaginary line down the middle of your body, dividing the front and back portions of your body, and bring your awareness to the front of your body. Do you notice any body part that is letting you know it's there? Just notice, without judgment. Are your toes tense, shoulders tight, hips uncomfortable? Maybe you feel a twinge in your belly. Maybe you feel totally at ease and peaceful. Again, just notice. Now, ask your body, "Do you have any wisdom for me?" See what your body answers. It may beckon you to shift your weight, soften the tension in your neck or release the muscles that are tightly squeezing the bones in your feet. It may tell you to eat breakfast earlier than 11 a.m.; lie differently at night; or carry your baby, briefcase or bags on your other side for a while. You may get the message from your body to schedule a massage or call a professional to assist in your healing. You may get a confirmation that your recent health choices are working quite well for you. Next, bring your awareness to the back section of your body and repeat your scan from head to toe. If you like, you can repeat this scan by sectioning the right and left sides of your body or top and bottom. The idea is to isolate a section and rest your thoughts there, do a scan, feel and observe the sensations and then ask your body to guide you. When you are ready, gently open your eyes.

3

Actively Participate in Your Health

○ ○

Health is the willingness to participate in what's going on.

—*Christiane Northrup, M.D.*

Take a minute to think of the last time you were sick or injured. What did you do to accelerate your healing? Depending on the nature of the illness or injury, prescription drugs may have been an essential part of the healing process. Did you take them as prescribed? Did you take them longer than necessary? If you were taking antibiotics, were you sure to finish the entire cycle of pills? Were there homeopathic options to consider? Were you including high-quality nutritional supplements in your wellness plan? Did you put all your healing focus outside of you—on the medicine or on the medical care providers? Did you envision yourself healing quickly?

I know a story about a woman who walked into a hospital room to visit her friend. When she asked her friend how she was feeling, the patient replied, "I don't know, the doctor hasn't come in yet."

In contrast, I have a different story. In 2004, I was sitting on a porch swing that collapsed, propelling me backward. My head violently made impact with the house. It was quite metaphorical at the time, as I felt the house "hit me on the head" while my husband and I were painfully discussing our upcoming divorce. I felt an excruciating pain in the back of my head and a sparking of electrical impulses shuddering from my spine through my limbs. My teeth momentarily clamped shut and I was understandably stunned.

After hours in the emergency room and many tests—all of which I insisted they show me the results of before I decided to approve the next test—the doctor came in to report the results of the CT Scan and MRI. He told me I did not have a brain bleed (which he had been concerned about), but I did have a pretty serious concussion. He then cleared his throat and looked at me quite seriously. "The tests also show you have cervical degenerative disease in your neck and this will only get worse at you get older." I returned his eye-to-eye contact and said firmly and simply, "No it won't." As I kept his gaze with such determination, he slowly began to smile and contritely replied, "Well, okay."

I then told him he didn't know what I did for a living or how I thought and that I personally had no plans for my head to begin drooping or for my neck to hurt more every year as I aged. I share this because if someone had pronounced this diagnosis to me decades ago, I would have been the perfect patient and a textbook case of someone with this condition. (I was in a nasty car accident in my twenties and suspect the initial damage to the cervical vertebrae had been done long ago. Just for the record, this wasn't the result of the porch swing accident.)

With the amazing advancements in the field of medicine, surrendering your power to a medical professional comes easily. Fortunately, many health care practitioners believe they work better when the person being treated feels powerful in choosing options for treatment. How do you heal? Do you let someone else choose for you with or without asking questions? Do you actively participate in your health?

Valuing your own inner healing process is essential. For example, if you're getting a cold, do you go to the store and buy the latest cold medicine and pop it down as you continue your busy pace? Or do you pause to nurture and treat your body to a warm bath, soothing herbal tea, and the comfort of your bed? If you are at home with small children and a warm bath sounds like a great fantasy, do you call a friend and ask for a bit of a respite, even an hour's worth? Do you moan and groan and tell everyone how terrible you feel, or do you consciously choose to acknowledge your illness but attempt to move through it with optimism?

Many years ago, an insightful family practitioner told me he could either give me some cold medicine and I would get better in seven days, or I could pamper myself, rest, and drink lots of fluids and get better in a week! Try observing (without judging) what you do the next time you become sick or injured. I am not suggesting that you should deny you are sick. I am not suggesting that you shouldn't seek appropriate medical care to partner in your healing. I am suggesting that *you* become the writer of this script. Practice loving self-care and self-appreciation—listen to your body's wisdom. What is this injury or illness telling you?

When practicing self-care it is important to remember to also pay attention to the more intimate parts of our body such as breasts and testicles. It is sad to consider that the fear we have created around breast cancer may lead to the belief that breasts are just malignancies waiting to happen. In addition to breast self-exams and recommended mammograms (or better yet, breast thermography), I say love your breasts: touch them, caress them, open your arms high and wide and create a morning stretch that sends an increased blood flow to that part of your body. (Actually, men have breasts too, although we usually call them the "chest.") When you're in the shower, lather up and caress, honor, and send love to that special part of your body that covers your heart—whether you have breasts or you've had a mastectomy. If you are a breast cancer survivor, touch, love, and caress the heart and chest space where your breasts once were or where your new breasts are. Your essence can never be surgically removed.

American society glorifies the female breasts as physical symbols of sexual pleasure, desire, and worth. But our own notions of sexual pleasure, desirability, and worth reside in our brains. Luckily for us, we have the amazing ability to control that part of our being, no matter what body part may be missing or wounded. Our minds are so powerful. Tap into that internal power daily and notice the peace that results.

Breast and testicular health is often spoken about in whispers. These precious parts of the body don't need to be any more secret than the heart or lungs. We need to take time to care for all parts of the body during our life's journey.

Testicular health is of particular concern to men between the ages of 15 and 39, the typical age for testicular cancer to occur. Testicular cancer has one of the highest cure rates of all cancers so don't wait to get a lump checked. Be sure to seek medical care immediately after discovering a lump. Early detection provides many healing options. Self-exams for lumps can be done with a positive attitude and pleasuring stroke of the hand. And, men, I don't think I'm telling you anything new about the pleasure of touch in this special area! Feel free to touch your testicles and say, "I love my testicles! I love my testicles!" And if you have an un-descended testicle or had one surgically removed, love and touch the beautiful skin of your scrotum.

Keeping your mind filled with healthy thoughts and taking appropriate medical action when necessary is a powerful combination. When you actively participate in your health, you will see amazing results.

Questions to Support You in Implementing the Ideas in This Chapter

1. Call to mind the last time you were sick or injured. What did you do to support or accelerate your healing?

2. How did you take part in any medical decisions that needed to be made? Did you ask questions and explore any choices?

3. What activities do you do to create a healthier physical body? Would you like to add an activity that would further enhance your health?

4. Do you frequently choose healthy foods that nourish you?

5. What one thing would you like to commit to so you can more actively participate in your health?

4

Observe How You Talk to Your Body

○ ○

The more we accept ourselves, the more fully we experience the world.

—Stephen Levine

How do you talk to your body? If you like, just observe your self-talk as you go about the day today. Will you hear a critical voice saying, "I'm so fat, I hate my thighs, look at those wrinkles, I hate my belly, I am so tired, I hate this mole on my neck, these veins are ugly, I always get sick, my arthritis is acting up again …"? You get the picture. Well, the immune system gets the picture too and does a great job of being quite the creative artist in your body. Your immune system actually responds to your thoughts. Yes, really! It's now a proven fact.

Candace Pert, Ph.D., has done significant research to identify a substance in the body called neuropeptides. These chemicals are released in the body with every emotion and they are actually measurable. Any time we feel various emotions, our neuropeptides can detect them and can actually record and store them on a cellular level. Our emotions truly affect our physical bodies. The good news is: our pleasant emotions create positive cellular responses. And that is something good to remember.

For an incredible example of how our emotions and thoughts profoundly influence the body, read Jill Bolte Taylor's book, *My Stroke of Insight*. Dr. Taylor is a Harvard-trained neuroanatomist who, in 1996, experienced a rare form of stroke that affected the left hemisphere of her brain. She combines her brilliant training as a neuroanatomist with the recounting of her personal experience of her recovery from this stroke. She boldly discusses how we can consciously influence how our brain chemistry is affected by our thoughts, feelings, and reactions to life events.

Simply observing the little inner voice that criticizes you can be the first step in becoming aware of the thoughts that flow through your mind. This observing self is often referred to as the "witness"—the loving, non-judgmental voice that simply watches and listens. I love to call it the "observette," a term my friend Donna coined years ago.

You can create a higher level of wellness consciousness simply by lovingly observing your self-defeating thoughts. Then instead of saying, "My thighs are so fat," you might affirm, "My thighs are toning up and looking better every day." Observation leads you back to that intentional part of your thinking. If you say an affirming statement, intend for it to happen, and take action on that intention, you'll soon find yourself making choices that create positive change.

I do want to point out that this idea isn't a magical fix. You can't tone your thighs by sitting on the couch, eating cake and ice cream every night chanting, "My thighs are toning up and looking better every day." Sorry, life doesn't work like that. Take action!

In his inspirational work, *The Four Agreements,* Don Miguel Ruiz suggests being "impeccable with your word." I understand this agreement to mean that we not only speak our word of truth to others, but that our self-talk also benefits from a truthful tone. Learning to speak lovingly to yourself holds a higher level of truth and integrity than talking to yourself in a self-deprecating manner. Observe how you talk to yourself and make choices that will allow your self-appreciation and your wellness wisdom to expand.

Three Suggestions to Support You in Implementing the Ideas in This Chapter

1. Lovingly observe how you talk to or about your body this week. Become a non-judging "observette." Just notice. Note: You may find yourself becoming increasingly aware of how

others talk about their aches and pains and bodies. It's best to just observe this too, with love and non-judgment.

2. If you find your inner voice is critical, stop and take a deep breath, then decide if you are ready to reframe that thought. For example, the initial thought "My thighs are so flabby and out of shape" might be re-framed to "My thighs are beginning to tone up since I started to take the steps more than the elevator!"

3. Make loving observations a fun practice until you find you no longer, or rarely, think or speak self-deprecating or un-flattering thought or words. Eventually, you will have fewer of these thoughts to weed out of your mental garden!

5

Nourish the Body/Mind

○ ○

I acknowledge that this choice to eat is a fundamental act of
love and nourishment, a true celebration of my existence.
—*Marc David*

Let's discuss self-nourishment first, before talking about fruits and vegetables. Self-nourishment involves those things you do to fill your body and your mind so you don't get depleted as you face life's everyday activities and challenges. Deepak Chopra, M.D., recognizing the powerful connection between the two, often refers to the *body/mind*. The term body/mind describes the inseparable connection between the body and the mind.

Many people have learned to hold back from nourishing themselves, allowing negative self-talk to eat away at their wholeness. Do you feed your body/mind with negative talk? Would you like to stop that inner dialogue? Not an easy thing to do, you say? Maybe not, but why sabotage yourself? We can choose to better nourish ourselves and re-program our minds with more loving thoughts and beliefs. Soon we can transform these beliefs into what Chopra refers to as *knowings*. Knowings can take us a step deeper into a place where we freely tap into our inner wisdom, where we don't need to change a belief anymore because we simply know it to be true.

Are you willing to give up the sabotaging beliefs that have kept you stuck? Over time we may become quite comfortable with these beliefs and we might not want to detach from them. They're painful, but they are familiar. We cling to them, clutching them to us like a special toy. We shine up this toy (our belief) and don't want anyone to pull it away from us. Many of these beliefs caused us to create brilliant survival tactics when we were only four or five years old. Beliefs and responses that worked successfully for years may now be outdated and ineffective. What a relief it can be to release them.

Many people have chosen to tap the strength and power within themselves to change affirming beliefs into knowings. Set your intention. Focus on the things you can do *today* to provide your own self-nourishment and then take action. Don't wait for your mother to stop criticizing you or your father to love you or your partner to flatter you or your friends to make it okay. It's up to you.

What can you gain by shedding these beliefs? Oh, so much. It's hard to heal this aspect of your life if you are unwilling to surrender the belief that fuels the behavior. Once we understand how much power our mind has over our body, it's almost impossible to stay stuck. How good is your relationship with your mind? Strive to make it stronger and begin to look for nourishing and flourishing results.

Before moving on to discussing the actual foods we eat, it might be good to take a moment to look at what we put on our plate. Not our dinner plate, but our "to do list" plate. Elizabeth Gilbert, best-selling author of one of my favorite books, *Eat, Pray, Love*, shared a statement during an interview with Oprah Winfrey that has had a powerful impact on me. She stated simply, "I am my best person when I have less on my plate." I instantly saw my metaphorical plate as having way too much stuff on it! There have been times when I have found myself jumping from one activity to another, or spinning like a hamster with wild abandon on a wheel that wasn't really taking me anywhere. Sound familiar?

Next I brought to mind an image of my dinner plate and smiled, realizing how I have gradually and pleasantly made a shift from eating more at lunchtime (when food digests better) and less at dinner. Then I thought about my emotional plate and observed that I am getting better at watching my emotions come and go and getting less attached to them. And finally, I conjured up an image of my spiritual plate and felt full of blessings, love, and gratitude—and felt quite satisfied.

I want to be the best person I can be, as I nourish my body/mind. I plan to say "yes" when I mean yes, "no" when I mean no, and to be kinder to myself by dancing off the hamster wheel and keeping things more simple and meaningful.

What's on your plate? Are you happy with your choices? It's a great time to assess whether you want to continue at the pace you have chosen, or whether you want to mindfully get in there and make a few adjustments. Hmm, I just realized that if you slip an "e" into the word "pace" it becomes "peace." Are you at peace with your choices?

Now let's talk about the actual foods you eat. How many servings of fruits and vegetables did you eat yesterday? If it appeals to you, put this book down and go to the kitchen or corner store and bring back an apple or carrot to eat while you finish reading this section.

Most people are well aware of the research that shows the connection between eating more fruits and vegetables and lowering the risk of cancer, heart disease, and other common illnesses. The recommendation to eat "five a day" seems simple enough, yet many people struggle to include one or two servings in their daily choices. Simply adding one more fruit or vegetable into your food choices today is a good place to start.

I no longer use the word "diet" in my language, after someone pointed out that the first three letters of that word aren't very inspiring! I like to say "live-it" when talking about a food plan. It seems easier to make wiser choices when we aspire to live rather than merely to avoid dying. So, please stop the guilt trips and the negative self-talk about eating and begin to observe the words you use to describe food. "Sinfully delicious" just doesn't taste the same to me as "gloriously delicious." Your body can digest the latter easier and you may find yourself enjoying your food without guilt.

Counting grams of fat, tracking calories, and looking at numbers on a scale can often keep quality nourishment at bay. Obviously, if you have a health concern that requires you to avoid or limit certain foods, then it's prudent to carefully check labels. But I suggest throwing away the scale unless every time you step on it you somehow get a jolt of joy! Otherwise, it can be an act of sabotage and can keep you stuck. If your daily food selections involve a variety of healthy carbohydrates (fresh fruits and vegetables, beans, high fiber grains) a good source of protein, and good fats (like olive oil, fish oil, or salmon), your eating can be a healthy pleasure. What a guilt-free and nourishing gift to the mind, body, and spirit!

Balance is another thing to keep in mind when making food choices. (We'll explore balance in the next chapter.) You can enjoy having a piece of chocolate, a cookie, or a piece of cake now and then, unless you have a medical condition that contraindicates this, such as diabetes.

Have you heard of the 80/20 rule? It suggests choosing really healthy foods at least 80% of the time. Here's one example. Not long ago I was standing in a grocery store line behind a woman who was asking the check-out clerk which bag of candy she should buy. She had a bag of Weight Watchers candy in one hand and strawberry Twizzlers in the other. The woman then turned to me to ask my advice, hoping I might add insights on calories, sugar, and grams of fat. I simply asked her, "Which candy would you REALLY enjoy?" The hand with the Twizzlers shot high in the air. "Then buy those," I said, "And take three breaths before you begin eating, say a little prayer, and then absolutely enjoy each bite!" I then gently suggested she might consider buying blueberries or fresh strawberries too so she could have healthier options when the sweet cravings hit. The Twizzlers, in my opinion, would fall into the "20" part of the 80/20 rule.

Food is to nourish *and* to be enjoyed! Be aware of refined sugars though, as they seem to "refine" our ability to know when to stop eating them.

Speaking of sugar, let's discuss the nourishing concept of low-glycemic eating. If you crave carbohydrates or sugar, you are not alone. Carbs are not bad; in fact our bodies need carbohydrates like fruits, vegetables, whole grains, and beans. It's the easily digestible carbs like white bread, white rice, sugars, sodas, and highly-processed foods that cause cravings and can result in weight gain, heart disease, and Type 2 diabetes. We are learning it's really not fat that makes you fat; it's too much sugar (and hidden sweeteners) that makes you fat.

As you can see in the list above, all carbohydrate foods are not created equal. Various carbs cause our bodies to behave quite differently after we eat them. The glycemic index, or GI, is a tool that makes it easier to choose foods that keep our blood sugar levels steady, and thus help to prevent heart disease and diabetes. Eating foods with a low glycemic index (55 or under) is also a major key to sustaining weight loss. Glycemic load (GL) is another concept to consider. It takes into consideration the quantity of the food consumed. Multiple Web sites provide detailed lists of carbohydrates and their corresponding GI and GL numbers.

When we consume high-glycemic foods, it causes an over-stimulation of the release of insulin. Because of how insulin works in our body, the more high-glycemic foods we eat, the more we crave. Have you noticed? Medical studies show that over 85% of the carbohydrates consumed in the Western world are foods that have a high-glycemic value. That means, if you eat a high-glycemic meal, you feel hungry again about an hour after you eat because your blood sugar has dropped. So you reach for another cookie or bagel and your blood sugar spikes again. You feel great for a while until your blood sugar drops once again. So then you eat, not because of a lack of will power, but because every cell in your body is screaming for another hit of sugar. You can stop this roller coaster and reset the body at a cellular level to break the cycle by eating three low-glycemic meals a day and having two low-glycemic snacks in between. Dr. Ray Strand's *Healthy for Life* book is a great source of detailed information on this topic.

Along with being familiar with blood sugar levels and the glycemic index of foods, it might be wise to have your vitamin D levels checked. It seems we've been taught to fear the sun so much that researchers are now finding a correlation between low levels of vitamin D and a list of degenerative diseases. In a review article published in *The New England Journal of Medicine,* Dr. Michael Holick explores the nature of vitamin D deficiency and concludes it to be one of the most commonly unrecognized medical conditions. His research reports that this deficiency is a factor in developing osteoporosis as well as other serious illnesses such as heart disease, cancer, infectious diseases, and autoimmune diseases. Dr. Holick's book, *The Vitamin D Solution,* "sets a new standard in health and wellness that I believe will change the face of medicine as we know it," according to Dr. Andrew Weil. Check with your care provider to see if he or she recommends optimal levels (experts are suggesting 40-100 ng/ml) of vitamin D.

Speaking of vitamin D, I recommend choosing supplements that meet Good Manufacturing Practice (GMP) standards. Companies that use GMP choose pharmaceutical grade (rather than food grade) manufacturing processes. High quality supplements add to your healthy food choices and are an important investment in your health. Even if we eat all organically grown food, it is still important to supplement. Our soil has been depleted of its original richness and toxins have invaded our precious earth. My grandparents didn't need to supplement but today it's a different world. Even the American Medical Association reversed its long-time stance on supplements in its 2002 recommendation that all adults take multivitamins. So eat wholesome foods and take your vitamins.

Not all vitamins are created equal. One source I highly recommend is a study commissioned by the Canadian parliament. The results were published in the *NutriSearch Comparative Guide to Nutritional Supplements*. The fourth edition of this independent guide, written by Lyle MacWilliam, M.Sc., F.P., compares over 1,500 nutritional products in North America for quality, bioavailability, potency, purity, and safety.

Another great resource is the Health Assessment and Advisor link at www.usana.com. You'll find recommendations based on your own needs and lifestyle. Pages 740-41 in Dr. Christiane Northrup's 4th edition (2010) of *Women's Bodies, Women's Wisdom* contains a succinct list of tips for choosing supplements. After checking these resources to see how your supplements are rated, I would use your intuition to guide you to the next steps. Your body contains much wisdom and I love recommending combining "outside" experts with your own "inside" expert.

If you are looking for other quality resources to spark and sustain the goodness in your own eating habits, I highly recommend Marc David's book, *The Slow Down Diet: Eating for Pleasure, Energy, & Weight Loss*. It is the single most valuable book I have ever read on this topic. It is not a diet based on restriction, but rather a supportive, well-researched, and soul-filled guide to understanding food, our choices, how we eat, and what we eat. David is a nutritionist with a master's degree in the psychology of eating and infuses his wisdom with many years of experience.

A great companion to Marc David's book is *Create the Body Your Soul Desires* by Drs. Karen Wolfe and Deborah Kern. These authors describe a buddy system that provides support for creating and energizing your eating plan. This concept of not having to venture alone has proven to be a powerful key to success in creating the body your soul desires. An added bonus is the way they address transforming self-limiting beliefs into empowering ones.

Enjoy what you eat, tune in to your wisdom, and be mindful of what truly nourishes your body/mind. Keep your food choices varied, fresh, unprocessed, and balanced. Eat mindfully, seek pleasure, make knowledgeable choices, and enjoy each bite.

Questions (and Answers) to Support You in Implementing the Ideas in This Chapter

1. Who is eating? Is it a calm, relaxed being, or a stressed out body in a rush? Is it a man or woman who remembers the voice of a family member criticizing them for food choices, or a person with loving awareness of how food can gently nourish the body and soul? You are the *who*. Bring your best, wisest, and highest self to the table.

2. What should you eat? Michael Pollan, author of *In Defense of Food*, advocates, "Eat food. Not too much. Mostly plants." I would add: eat organic and locally grown foods when possible, enjoy foods in season, keep sugar intake low, and stay away from artificial sweeteners. (Did you know that Aspartame has been re-branded as Amino Sweet? Yikes!) Avoid fatty foods, eat foods that are low-glycemic so your blood sugar stays stable, and choose a variety of color in each meal. Choose healthy protein sources. Complement your diet with pharmaceutical grade supplements. Follow the 80/20 rule, which suggests choosing really healthy foods at least 80% of the time. Remember, if your daily food selections involve a variety of fresh fruits and vegetables, a good source

of protein, high fiber grains, and good fats, your eating can be a pleasure. Know what good carbohydrates are: whole grains, fruits, vegetables, and beans. I am not an advocate of counting calories, grams of fat, or constantly getting on the scale—unless you get on the scale and a delightful voice calls out to remind you of the precious and beautiful being you are! Lighten up. Stop thinking restriction and focus on creating healthy food cravings instead.

3. Where should you eat? Or where shouldn't you eat? Do not eat standing at the kitchen sink, in front of your computer or TV, in the car, at your desk, or at fast food places. When possible, sit down at a table, even if you are eating alone. Individuals and families who create sacred meal times reap countless benefits.

4. When should you eat? Early and often! Start the day with a healthy breakfast that doesn't spike your blood sugar (typical culprits are a latte and muffin, orange juice and sugary cereals, or pastries). Skipping breakfast leads to weight gain, a drop in blood sugar, and other adverse effects on the metabolism. Eating three meals a day and having two low-glycemic healthy snacks between meals keeps your blood sugar and mood on an even track. Going long periods of time without eating actually can add weight because your body goes into fight/flight mode, thinks it's starving, dumps more cortisol in your stomach, and slows your digestive system—creating more fat. Eating after 7 p.m. can result in what's been labeled "the sumo wrestler's diet" since your food hangs out in your stomach while you sleep, eventually adding extra pounds in the process.

5. Why should you eat? For health, energy, and pleasure.

6. How should you eat? Mindfully. Taking three breaths (and maybe saying a prayer) before each meal sets the tone for a nourishing break in the day. Setting the dinner table with flowers, candles, good dishes (what are we saving them

for anyway?), and cloth napkins is nurturing and calming. People who ban complaining from mealtime conversations tend to digest their food better. Taste your food! Sprinkle it with the spice of love. Savor each bite.

6

Gently Seek Balance and Joy

○ ○

Your deepest presence is in every small contracting or expanding, the two as beautifully balanced and coordinated as bird wings.

—Rumi

The concept of balance is key in many areas of wellness including time management and nourishment choices. Balancing time with care—care for yourself and for others—may sometimes feel like a tightrope walk. You may want to choose a day to focus on balance in just one area of your life. Gently observe your patterns and notice where you feel in sync or where you feel off balance. You may want to ask yourself, "Am I overdoing anything? Am I avoiding or ignoring something that might be affecting my sense of balance? What would make me feel more balanced?" Then commit to making small changes that will lead you back into a more centered place.

When choosing foods, I am usually aware that if I have chocolate in the house (okay, it's not *if* I have chocolate—I ALWAYS have chocolate in the house), I need to be sure to reach for the fruit or veggies more often than I do the chocolate. Because when I do, I can *choose* chocolate and really take time to savor and enjoy its pleasurable taste. (Please note that I have just paused to savor the piece of organic dark chocolate that's in my mouth as I write this paragraph!) That's one way of balancing my food choices; and it feels right to me.

Simply observing when we're off balance can actually help us in regaining our balance. Observation is a powerful tool. If we remember to take the time to tune in to ourselves, we can become more aware of when we're off balance physically, emotionally, mentally, or spiritually. We can also gently seek to get back into balance if we are awake and aware of our choices.

If you are willing, pick one area in your life where you feel off balance. Then take a moment to write a commitment statement that would focus your attention toward balance. For example, if you notice you are running in all directions much of your day, your commitment statement might be, "I commit to taking more time each day to be silent and still."

As you create more balance in your life, you may want to add a big dollop of joy too. In fact, you may want to be very conscious and intentional about seeking joy, because sometimes we forget. Sometimes our minds are scurrying off into wild places and it's important to put a good, joy-filled spin on what we are thinking.

" . . . for there is nothing either good or bad, but thinking makes it so." This famous line from Shakespeare's *Hamlet* presents the idea that we can choose our thoughts. Although one might easily argue that some things really *are* bad, the idea that we can put our own spin on our thoughts is quite powerful. We can use that power to create intentional joy or distressing moments.

Here's a beautiful example. My son, Zack, is an amazing musician. (Written like a proud mom, I admit.) Not long ago, when he was playing at an outdoor venue, a five-year-old girl came up to him and asked, "What makes the music sound so beautiful?" Zack tenderly replied, "You do."

That's it! That's the secret to creating a joyful life! What makes anything appear to be good or bad, beautiful or ugly, distressing or joyful? YOU DO! You have the power to choose your thoughts and to put an overlay of joy around them when you can.

As mentioned in Chapter 1, we have over 60,000 thoughts a day. Many of them are the same as the day before. It has become increasingly clear to me that how we think has a huge impact on our everyday happiness and wellness. We get to cultivate powerful choices or, by default, let the old tapes of disempowerment or victim-hood play over and over in our heads. Sometimes our brains get so depleted of serotonin and dopamine because of chronic or steady stressors and medical support is needed. "Thinking happy thoughts" would be too simplistic a remedy in these cases. The idea of seeking balance and joy wouldn't even be on our radar screen.

The Christmas season of 2009 was a gigantic practice session for my thinking and seeking balance and joy. I spent two weeks on the east coast where the record-breaking December snowstorm became my wildly unpredictable travel agent. After spending four days in the Toronto area, I had awakened to beautiful weather the morning of December 20 and attempted to print my boarding passes for flights to Charlottesville. Imagine my surprise when I discovered the airport was closed due to heavy snow! I remember being quite excited and anxious to see my children, grandchildren, and friends there, but for some reason I remained calm. I became aware that I only had control of my thoughts, not the airports or the weather. So, I was starting out calm, balanced, and joyful.

The next ten days provided me with numerous opportunities to either get really angry, frustrated, or unbalanced—or to choose thoughts that would redirect that unpleasant energy into joyful thoughts. So many unpredictable things happened that I felt like there was a game being played in my head. I became an "observette" to my thoughts and surroundings, more than ever before. I only came close to losing it twice—out of a dozen great opportunities to do so.

The first time was the morning of December 21. I had been standing in line for three hours at the Charlotte airport in North Carolina, where they were dealing with thousands of stranded travelers from the weekend storm. I had been re-routed there the day before since I couldn't fly into Charlottesville, Virginia. It actually turned out to be a great blessing since I was able to be with my younger sister on her birthday. Hmmm, it seemed God had bigger plans!

But, getting back to why I was about to fall into a heap on the airport floor . . . I was tired, hungry, and had to go to the bathroom—not a pretty trio of needs to have while confined in an airport line. At some point I realized I was going to miss the morning flight because of the chaos surrounding me, and I did. It was now 10 a.m. and I was re-booked on a 10 p.m. flight and given standby boarding passes for three overbooked flights to attempt to board during the day. It took me longer than a few minutes to switch my very un-balanced and distressed thoughts to joy. I have forgiven myself for the unkind thoughts that I was really, really trying hard not to direct toward any airline employee. They had had a tough weekend. Plus, several of my family members work for the airlines . . .

I met people who had missed funerals, weddings, and cruises. I was greatly missing precious moments with my children and grandchildren. It seemed others had more reasons to get upset than I did. The observation of thoughts continued. I eventually landed in snow-bound Charlottesville.

The other time I almost lost it was my last day in Virginia. We had just pulled my two suitcases on a sled about one-third of a mile down the drive in order to reach my friend's car. My friend Phyllis' long driveway was still icy and she couldn't park close to her house. I fell twice (head first) and the sled tipped over several times. Amazingly, I didn't lose it then. I kept laughing and wishing I had a camera. (Note: I had had a blast pulling the suitcases on the sled down the mile-long driveway nine days earlier, three days after an unexpected stay at the Holiday Inn due to the two feet of white stuff in a land of little snow plowing! But now I was heading to the airport and knew the plane wouldn't wait for me.)

No, I started to fall apart after we loaded the luggage into the car and I was about a half mile from where the driveway connected with the road. I lost it when the car slowly, uncontrollably, and gracefully slid off the icy drive and turned sideways to become lodged in the field of snow. The car remained stuck there for days, as the Blue Ridge Mountains reflected its beauty off the windshield. I said the four-letter word for "poop" out loud and spent about ten seconds (or was it 10 minutes?) in panic and frustration. Balance? Joy? At the time, they were nowhere to be found.

I was about to miss my plane and I was really, really ready to get home. Then I chose—really consciously chose—to change my thinking. My thought turned from frustration to a calm, "Hmm, I wonder what's going to happen next?" Things were clearly out of my control and I could go with the flow in the snow or fight and struggle and be quite miserable. I decided to intentionally seek joy.

While Phyllis scurried back to her house to call a neighbor to help dig us out, I dragged one of my bags up closer to the country road and prayed for the little patch of cell phone reception that I can sometimes get there on a clear day. Success! I was able to reach my son who lives 30 minutes away. Zack sped to my rescue and arrived (sped being the key word here) 20 minutes later. It seemed God wanted me to have my son take me to the airport that day and I was beyond grateful that I didn't miss my flight. It was another lesson in choosing thoughts to be open to something better, and to wait for the miracle that could occur.

After arriving safely at the quaint Charlottesville airport, the ticket agent asked how my day was going so far. I refrained from hysterical laughter and instead gave a brief account of the trip with its many detours and delays. I then asked her if, by chance, there were any first class seats available on my connecting flight out of Charlotte for my five-and-a-half-hour flight back to Seattle. At this point, I was ready to pay for comfort and ease! I was seeking intentional joy! She put me on the standby list for first class and told me if they *did* have a seat open up, I wouldn't have to pay extra upgrade costs. A seat didn't appear but the thought that she tried *almost* negated the three-hour wait in line I'd experienced at the Charlotte airport the week earlier. Bless those airline employees!

Allow the expanding and contracting of life's activities to find a gentle place of balance in all areas of your life. Observe when you are in balance and when you are not. Be open to seeking balance and intentional joy.

Three Tips to Support You in Gently Seeking
Balance and Intentional Joy

1. Stop and breath. Feel what you are feeling and then take another deep breath. (You can even say "poop" if you have to!)

2. Observe what comes next as you take positive steps to make something different happen. Choose a thought that makes you feel better than you do right now—even if it's just a little bit better.

3. Be grateful. Look for and revel in the miracles that follow.

7

Honor the Body/Mind Temple

○ ○

Here in this body are sacred rivers: here are the sun and
moon as well as all the pilgrimage places . . . I have not
encountered another temple as blissful as my own body.

—*Saraha*

"I have not encountered another temple as blissful as my own body."
What a glorious statement! That's one to post on the refrigerator door
or bathroom mirror. In my opinion, the body/mind temple contains the
sacred as much as any temple, mosque, or church.

Once we begin to understand and believe the depth of connection
between the body and mind (as described in Chapter 5), we realize they
team up to offer a sacred and wondrous dynamic duo. If we honor our
mind with positive thoughts and images we may be more likely to treat
our physical body as the temple it is. And when we add a healthy dose
of a loving heart, the temple glows.

For some of us, this may mean a real rewiring of our current way of
thinking. We might need to dig deep and unearth the beliefs that have
kept our bodies stuck in a pattern of un-temple-like thinking. Society
has profoundly affected the way we think about our physical bodies.
The media continues to flaunt images of men and women models with
airbrushed perfect faces and bodies that don't really exist. It often sets
us up for failure and causes some people to overeat, undereat, to not care
what they eat, or to work out at a frenetic and unhealthy pace.

What *one* thing can you do today to honor your unique physical body? It can be something as simple as pausing now to stretch your arms to the heavens and recognize that the ability to change a habit resides within the body/mind attached to those arms.

What beliefs that no longer serve you might need to be thrown out of your life? Write them down and then burn the paper. Use the flame to ignite new thoughts in you, thoughts that know the truth of who *you* really are. It seems so simple and yet it is not always easy. Yet, it doesn't have to be so hard either. Wouldn't you rather change unhealthy beliefs and decrease the pain and anguish?

Questions to Support You in Going Deeper
Into Honoring the Body/Mind Temple

1. What one thing can you do today to honor your unique physical body?

2. What un-loving beliefs about your body/mind temple are you willing to release?

3. What do you have to gain from releasing them?

4. What attribute of your body or mind do you love most?

5. What action steps are you willing to take today to deepen your belief that the body/mind temple is a glorious place to treasure?

8

Know God

○ ○
I turn to the Presence of God at the center of my being and
it is here that I discover the nature of the Good which must
and does reside in the back of all people and events.
                                        —*Ernest Holmes*

The spiritual component of wellness is highly individual, as each of us can choose to know God and create our spiritual practice through the lens of our own religious, spiritual, and cultural beliefs. We call God a variety of names: Spirit, Jesus Christ, Allah, Krishna, Father, Father-Mother, Buddha, Higher Power, El-Shaddai, Jehovah, Tao, and All-That-Is. We may know the Divine to be masculine, feminine, both, or neither. Some people choose not to believe in God. This chapter speaks to those who have God or (insert whatever name you use) in their lives.

Knowing (not just believing) that God is always with me has changed my life dramatically in recent years. The Greek philosopher Empedocles said, "The nature of God is a circle of which the center is everywhere and the circumference is nowhere." God is so huge! Now I understand that there is "no place where God is not." I now recognize that God wants my path of wellness—and yours—to be a glorious path.

For many, envisioning a God up in heaven offers a profound solace. Others see the essence of God reflected in the sunsets, sunrises, flowers, oceans, mountains, moon and stars, in children, and in each other.

Whenever and however you connect with the God you know, you have the opportunity to find a sense of peace, joy, and well-being that nourishes the soul.

Spiritual wellness involves our perception of meaning and purpose in life. It relates to how we integrate our actions with our beliefs and values. Spiritual wellness considers our faith journey and how we live in relation to harmony, compassion, and peace. No matter where you may be on your journey, there are avenues that can lead to a greater understanding of your life's purpose.

I have found that when I take the time to quiet my chattering mind and consciously listen to God, profound shifts happen in my life. My moments are more full, the people I meet feel more loving, and the tasks I perform have more purpose. When I am feeling separate from God (even though I know I can't really be separate because God is always present—but sometimes I forget), then I often get into trouble as my thinking becomes cloudy and I revert to the "poor me" story. Since what I focus on expands, the poor me can get really drained. So, if I focus on the woes presented on the evening news, I then quickly take a dive into fearful thinking and can easily feel down. Instead, I have learned that an alternate way of watching the news is to see it as an opportunity to pray. What an amazing shift happens when I turn my attention to God.

However you choose to connect with God is highly personal. Your connection may deepen through prayer, meditation, ritual, churches, chapels, synagogues, and mosques, or through a walk in nature. Dedicating time to your own spiritual growth is an integral part of wellness. What one thing could you do today that would help you to know God more?

Steps to Take If You Want to Get to Know God Better

1. Create quiet time each day. You can start by taking just one minute before you get out of bed. Then gradually add to this precious ritual or practice as you begin your day. Some people like to light a candle, read from a holy text, play spiritual music, or just quietly breathe. Pick something that works for you. Treasure and protect that time. Quiet

time for some may come, if only briefly, after you fall into bed after a long day. Breathe. Open your heart. Listen. God's there.

2.   Explore places where you feel closest to God and hang out there when you can. Examples include but are not limited to: churches, synagogues, mosques, chapels, temples, beaches, forests, mountains, with your family, or in your garden.

3.   Take time to talk with God. And then, take time to listen to God. You'll love the results. Praying doesn't change God—it changes us.

4.   Remember that what you focus on expands. So, focusing on God can provide a greater awareness of the Divine in your daily life. This doesn't mean you need to become a monk or priestess! It just means that the more you look for good and God, the more you'll discover both.

5.   What, if any, rituals or prayers from your childhood hold special meaning for you? Add or create a new practice if you like. Enjoy reading the next chapter for more ideas.

9

Pray and Meditate

○ ○

In the solitude of your mind are the answers to all of your questions about life. You must take the time to ask and listen.

—Bawa Mahaiyaddeen

However you choose to pray, you will deepen the communication between you and the Divine. I view praying as a reverent act of deeply communing with or talking to God. The message goes out as if we were talking to someone on the phone. I view meditation as listening to God via a heavenly phone—to recognize that voice we must be quiet so we might hear.

Declarative prayer is one of the many ways of communicating with God. With declarative prayer, you state that you accept the quality or thing you want in your life right now. An example would be, "I accept radiant health and wholeness." Until a few years ago, I had always prayed using the "Please God" begging method. Now I *assume* divine help and support. Everyone prays differently and I certainly believe God listens to us however we pray; but I really like this positive, trusting, affirming method and it has been extremely powerful in my life. I'm learning to give up a time line, to trust divine guidance. I'm also learning to give up being right about many things. And there are times when I still get down on my knees, sometimes weeping with a "Please God" at the beginning (and the end) of my prayer. God listens.

Some people love reading the Bible, the Koran, Bhagavad Gita, The Course in Miracles, or from the Vedic texts. Others enjoy poetry or philosophical readings to connect them to Spirit. You may find the prayers of your childhood to be soothing. Find what works best for you.

There's a beautiful meditation that I have found to be simple yet profound. It's from an ancient Hawaiian practice known as Ho'oponopono (meaning "to make right.") The words are simple and powerful: "I am sorry, please forgive me, I love you, I thank you." What's your favorite prayer?

In the early nineties, I had the honor of meeting monthly with my sangha "sisters" to enjoy dinner together, to listen to "what's up" for us, and to pray. (Sangha is a Sanskrit word that means "community.") We then shared our prayer requests for the month and agreed to pray for each other in between our meetings. Would a gathering of your own prayer community support your spiritual wellness?

I don't think God minds whether we declare what we most desire or simply ask for it. God is ever-present and knows you well, so praying the way that feels best for you will keep this part of your spiritual wellness sacred. The ritual of praying the rosary or reciting the Hebrew words that hold a place in your heart may be the way you connect and become closer with the Divine. If you are one of many seekers who yearn to heal wounds created by old religious beliefs, you may enjoy reading Joan Borysenko's *A Woman's Journey to God*. She offers inspiration to women and men who want to create new ways of prayer and connection to Spirit.

I've heard it said that prayer changes *us*, not God. It can be an empowering way of shifting so we know what the next best steps might be. Have you heard the saying, "Pray and move your feet"?

Meditation, a very ancient practice, is growing in popularity in our fast-paced western society filled to overflowing with cell phones, text messaging, Facebook, and BlackBerry technology. How interesting that meditation needs no expensive electronic equipment, just a quiet mind. Not too many years ago, if you lived in North America and told someone you were meditating they may have looked at you a little funny. Today, many people join meditation groups or classes and are aware that it is a practice done daily by many people worldwide.

Swiss-born psychiatrist, Elisabeth Kübler-Ross, author of the ground-breaking book *On Death and Dying* said, "Learn to get in touch with the silence within yourself and know that everything in this life has a purpose." It may seem intriguing to think we might need to get in touch with silence—it seems like such a simple act. Yet, for many of us, our mental chatter is in high gear during most of our waking hours. Taking the time to sit in silence opens up an avenue of peace that adds richness and deep wisdom to a spiritual practice. Take some time to listen, observe, and not judge the thoughts that pass through your head. Like clouds in the sky, thoughts pass by us and are replaced by new ones. Your gentle breath can guide you as you breathe in and breathe out.

As with prayer, many styles of meditating are available. Some individuals prefer to listen to their iPod or to CDs that provide guided meditations full of soothing words and images. You might enjoy listening to Karen Drucker's tender song *Morning Prayer* at the start of your day—it's one of my favorites. Other people meditate by sitting still or lying still in complete silence, quieting the mind of all thoughts. When a thought enters the mind, the idea is to notice it, observe it and let it pass. You can say, "That's a thought," and watch it melt away. Eventually, the noisy mind becomes still and you have access to divine wisdom. That wisdom is always there, I believe, but it has a tough time getting through our constant, sometimes flood-like stream of thoughts.

How would your day be different if you started it with just five minutes of silence? Ten minutes? How would your day be different if you added one of the above suggestions to your spiritual practices? If you're interested in experiencing the simplicity of silence, you can try taking a walk alone or planning an hour to move in silence with no TV, computer, music, or cell phone.

Like prayer, meditation is a gift you give yourself. Talking to God, listening to God—what a high and holy conversation. I can just hear God saying, "Can you hear me now?"

What practices do you have in place that sooth your soul? As I have strengthened the spiritual dimension of my own wellness path, these seven spiritual activities and resources have added blessings to my spiritual wellness. Everyone defines "spiritual wellness" in their own way and I want to note that the following resources are not affiliated with any religion. I encourage you to explore which activities feel right (if any) for you to add to your own practices of spiritual wellness.

Seven Practices to Enhance Your Spiritual Wellness

1. Start your day with five minutes of inspirational reading, music, or meditation. I often begin my day with Karen Drucker's beautiful song, "Morning Prayer." (From her latest CD Songs of the Spirit IIII.)

2. End your day with your own thank-you prayers or by mentally listing ten things you were grateful for that day.

3. Consider learning about the powerful Hawaiian practice called Ho'oponopono. It has simple, peaceful, and poignant lines: Dear God (Or whatever you call the Divine) I am sorry. Please forgive me. I love you. And I thank you. You may want to Google "Ho'oponopono" to explore resources that appeal to you.

4. Listen to healing music that sooths your soul. My favorite is the music to support the "healing stream" practice created by Bruno Groening (www.bruno-groening.org). This free music is available by clicking on "download" and then "music." My personal favorite is an instrumental entitled, "II Gitarre 2."

5. Subscribe to a daily message that uplifts your spirit. Abraham-Hicks Publications (www.abraham-hicks.com) has a daily quote I read at the start of my day. The top corner of their banner says, "You are loved. All is well." If I read nothing else, it's a great reminder that makes me smile each morning.

6. Create or discover a daily affirmation or short prayer that inspires and directs your day. Gay Hendricks shares what

he calls the "Ultimate Success Mantra" in his empowering book, *The Big Leap*. "I expand in abundance, success, and love every day, as I inspire those around me to do the same." I love this affirmation since it includes others too.

7. Find ways to access the healing power of love. If it calls to you, check out Robert G. Fritchie's work through the World Service Institute (www.worldserviceinstitute.org). This organization teaches people how to apply Divine Love as a healing energy to amplify spiritual wellness.

10

Live!

○ ○

I would rather be ashes than dust! I would rather that my spark should burn out in a brilliant blaze than it be stifled by dry rot. I would rather be a superb meteor, every atom of me in magnificent glow, than a sleepy and permanent planet. The proper function of man is to live, not to exist. I shall not waste my days in trying to prolong them. I shall use my time.

—Jack London

In 1998, my sister Cindy was diagnosed with twelve large and inoperable brain tumors. She was told she had two weeks to two months to live. She wasn't quite ready to go after two months and lived for three more, soaking up a lifetime of living in those five precious months. Cindy often used humor to get through her final days. About a month before she passed away, she looked me in the eye and said, "Susan, I think this is just all in my head!" We giggled and giggled, and then we cried.

In the few short months after her diagnosis at age 44, Cindy taught me to live my life more fully each day and to have more courage and less fear. I gained a new level of strength from being in her presence during those final weeks. One particular example was when she asked me and our other sister, Beth, to take her to the cemetery to see where she would be buried. We stood by her side as she said a solemn prayer over her own gravesite. How awesome it was to witness her strength and courage as she prepared to leave her children, grandchildren, family, and friends.

She also taught me not to waste a moment. Every day after her diagnosis with brain cancer, she would open her eyes and be so thrilled to still be alive that she would say, "Thank you, God, I get another day!" When she told me this it brought tears to my eyes and it made me feel like kicking myself for taking any day for granted. During the months of Cindy's illness, I would attend committee meetings at the university where I worked and observe people getting so upset about things they couldn't control, just like I had often done. All of these things seemed incredibly insignificant compared to the fact that my sister couldn't control what was happening, as her brain tumors grew larger each day. My perspective has been forever altered. My stressors have decreased dramatically. I awaken each morning thanking God for a new day.

Cindy's death gave me the gift of valuing each day as if it were my last. The petty grievances I had flew out the window. The irritation of waiting in the checkout line at the grocery store became insignificant. The traffic jams became just traffic. Life became so much easier.

My mother, father, and sister all died within five years of each other and it became too overwhelming to mark the anniversary of their deaths in the summer months of every year. So, I have reframed things to acknowledge "Heaven birthdays" instead. Heaven birthdays alter the concept of the "anniversary of a death" into the remembrance of a "celebration of life." It's a day to recall the joyful times and to call to mind the very best memories of a loved one's life. It is a way to place the focus on the life, rather than the death. This practice has done much to keep the value in my days and lightness in my spirit.

As we live our lives, we also need to find a way to truly live after we have lost someone close to us. Dealing with the loss of a loved one is hard. And offering support to someone who has just experienced a painful loss comes without a guidebook.

My daughter has a dear friend from Denmark, named Julie. Molly asked me to write to her after Julie lost her younger brother, Joachim, following complications from an illness he contracted while he was traveling in Laos. I had met Julie during her visit to the States years ago and I shared her sorrow. I wrote the following e-mail letter to her. She wrote back to tell me that she had read my letter to her family and it provided comfort for them in those days immediately after the burial.

Julie and her family have given me permission to print the letter here, with the vision of it providing solace for others who have experienced profound loss.

December 9, 2009

Dear Julie,

Molly just wrote to tell me about your brother. This is a sadness beyond any other. I am so, so sorry for your loss.

I am no stranger to death so I know that there are no magic words. People around you sometimes might not know what to do or say. Everyone wants you to feel better immediately and you can't. Everyone wants to take away your pain and they can't. But, they can love you, as I do, as Molly does, and hold you safely in their hearts, as we both do.

There are a few things that may be helpful to know. The first is that the pain is so deep, as deep and vast as your love for your brother. So, pain is an honoring of him, in a way. And then it will be time for the pain to subside but it will come back from behind, unexpectedly, for a while. And then, over time (and grief takes as long as it takes . . .) the pain will be replaced by a gentle knowing of the love and the memories and it will not hurt like it hurts now. I promise you that. And in time, the memories will overcome the pain like a sweet salve of peace. And, it will be okay not to be in pain so much. Some people want to cling to the pain all their life since they think that by letting it go it dishonors the memory. I don't believe that, personally. I think that the eventual peace that envelopes is the next natural step. Your brother will not want his death to be a heavy yoke around your neck all your life. He would rather his life be a garland of delightful, playful, and colorful flowers around your neck so that his undying love feels close to your heart. Love never dies.

And, in time, you may find yourself "talking" to his soul as if he were by your side. I absolutely, with every cell in my body, believe he will hear you. And, he may even answer you at times! My younger sister died in 1998. It was hard to make sense of it all; she was 44. But you only got to be with your brother for 24 years and that makes it even harder. And you didn't get to say goodbye and that is so sad too. So, when you're ready and if you want to, you can tell him goodbye by talking to his soul. He will hear you. He knows, (even more now than when he was on earth) that you loved him deeply. I know he feels the love of your entire family.

Please know that my heart surrounds your heart and my thoughts and prayers are with you and your family. I'm here for you if you want to write, yell, scream, or cry.

And, if it would make it better, I would send you all the peanut butter that Costco has.

I love you Julie.

Love,
Susan

Are you still experiencing the excruciating pain that comes from such a loss? I am so sorry for your loss, and trust that somehow in reading this little chapter that the salve of peace eases part of your grief. Grief takes as long as it takes and the living part of you will come alive again.

Are there things in your life that you put off doing until tomorrow? Are there people to forgive that would free you to feel lighter and happier? Do you want to expend energy on wondrous activities, or devote time to frustration and worry? Be a superb meteor! Go for it! Don't wait until tomorrow. LIVE! Live now. Now is all we have. And thank you, Cindy, for the gift you left me of treasuring each second of life.

Seven Healing Steps to Living After Loss

1. Allow yourself all the time you need to grieve, since grief takes as long as it takes. People around you may want to pull you out of it (because it's so hard for them to see you in such pain) and you can observe their concern with love. It's your loss, it's your sadness—not theirs. Be aware that each family member has his or her own timetable of moving through grief too.

2. If you find yourself almost ready to move forward to really *live* more fully but you're feeling blocked, ask yourself what belief you might need to give up by moving forward.

3. Take a moment to imagine what you might think about or where you might direct your energy if you no longer had the grief so present in your thoughts.

4. Once you find you are ready to move forward and release the cloak of grief that has been surrounding you, choose one nurturing thing to do that helps you get to the next step in your healing process.

5. When you are ready, you may want to consider doing something to help others. Gently stepping out of your own sadness and choosing to direct specific actions that have positive effects on others is a great way to shift your focus.

6. If you get stuck, and sometimes you will, don't hesitate to seek professional help. Find a therapist or healer that feels right for you... and this may mean experimenting a bit. One size therapist does not fit all. A recommendation from a friend may guide you but muster your intuition to really trust your own choice.

7. Live. Love. Laugh . . .when you are ready.

11

Create a Monthly Focus

What you focus on expands.

—Unknown

Each month you have an opportunity to create a monthly theme—a specific focus for expanding your wellness wisdom. For example, your theme for January could be movement (what some people call "exercise"). February could be love. March could be optimism. April could be financial freedom, and so on. Write your monthly focus on a piece of paper and place it on your refrigerator, on your computer or in your bathroom. Writing your focus and keeping it in a place where you can see it helps you to gather all your resources to move you closer toward that goal.

Here are some suggestions for your monthly themes:

Wellness	Beauty	Expansiveness
Wisdom	Clarity	Integrity
Nourishment	Peace	Movement
Laughter	Abundance	Personal Power
Love	Financial Freedom	Strength
Balance	Joy	Truth
Generosity	Ease	Worthiness
Order	Adventure	Forgiveness
Gratitude	Optimism	Pleasure

Keep it simple. If your theme is movement, choose the movement activity you want to add or expand into your weekly activities. But you might also take time to focus on how you walk, how you move into or out of a room, how you move your body when you get out of your car or into bed.

If your focus is on love, notice how filled up you feel when you give love in obvious ways or in gentle, subtle ways. If your focus is drinking more water, you may choose to drink more filtered water but you can also notice things like the feel of running water, the temperature of your shower or bath, the sound of the rain, or water sources around you. You can do all this just by placing your attention on water. This way, choosing to drink more water takes on an element of creativity and enjoyment that is something you want to do, not something you are forcing yourself to do.

You can enjoy the rejuvenation that often comes with the start of a new year each time a new month begins. You can also take time to start over or set intentions *any* time of the year. We don't need to have a calendar prompt us to create a new beginning.

Setting a monthly focus, creating intentions for the upcoming year, and clearing the slate to begin again are all things you can choose to do any day of the year. It's a wonderful way to nourish all aspects of you. What would you like to focus on this month?

Here are ten suggestions designed to propel you into action and keep you motivated as you create the best year ever—month by month. Each suggestion can inspire your choice of a monthly focus.

Ten Suggestions for the Best Year Ever

1. List your top five accomplishments for the previous 12 months and share them with a trusted friend. Clearing out the old year by recognizing the great things you have done paves the way for expansive opportunities in the New Year. And remember, you can choose to begin a new year today. After congratulating yourself for your accomplishments, make a list of five goals for the coming year. Beneath each

goal write two or three action steps that will move you closer to your goals. Mark these on your calendar to be sure you will remember them.

2. Make a list of the balances for your checking and savings accounts, retirement accounts, loans, and credit card balances. Many people have spent decades looking the other way and wishing, hoping or envisioning some miraculous windfall would land in their bank account, propelling them into financial ecstasy. Is this familiar to you? Then this can be your year for a serious turn-around. Take the emotion out of the numbers and get downright serious about paying off debt and spending and saving wisely. There are many books available to provide practical advice if you really are ready to take control of your financial well-being.

3. Remember—what you focus on expands. We have a choice of whether to concentrate on the doom and gloom of the nightly news or turn our attention toward our desires. This may mean limiting news-watching or watching or reading the news as if you were visiting from another planet. You can observe, with a sense of curiosity, how things are spun into disasters and note that the good news is rarely reported. You can concentrate on what you don't have, or on what you already have and want. It's that simple, and yet not always easy.

4. Take care and control of your health. Whatever your current health status, do all in your power to take control of your health. If you have a chronic or life-threatening illness, focus on how you want to feel or on the little successes. Avoid attaching the word "my" in front of an illness. When (and if) you are ready to do that, you will gain a sense of well-being that can't be measured through any blood test or MRI. Whatever level of health you have, amplify it. Eat well, think well, and move with pleasure. Think of yourself as always reaching a higher level of healthiness.

5. Never complain. Complaining is like praying for more of the same. It keeps you focused on what you don't want. Commit to 21 days without complaining and observe how much better you feel three weeks later. (There's more on this concept in Chapter 30.)

6. Love radically and intensely. Just do it—love intensely any chance you get. And in times of conflict or inner turmoil ask, "What would love do now?"

7. Forgive, forgive, forgive. This applies to forgiving yourself as well as others. Forgiving doesn't make a person's actions right, it frees you to move forward. How would you feel today if you gave yourself the blessings gained through forgiveness? Chapter 13 will provide you with more insights.

8. Be a pleasure-seeking missile. Become aware of what excites you to the core and if it's legal and doesn't hurt anyone, do it! Look for simple pleasures and create extravagant pleasures when you can.

9. Share what you have. Donate items to the thrift store, send money to your favorite charity, give money anonymously, give books to your local library or give your full attention as you listen to someone sharing his grief. Even when times may be economically challenging, keep the flow going by sharing what extra you do have to give. We all have something to give.

10. Thank God for all you have. Well, Amen to that! Happy New Year—beginning today!

12

Spend Money with Joy and Wisdom

○ ○

The more we learn to operate in the world based on trust in our intuition, the stronger our channel will be and the more money we will have.

—*Shakti Gawain*

Financial wellness is a big issue for many people. I believe this time of economic change will ultimately result in a redirection of the way we use and share our personal and natural resources. We have an opportunity to harness our collective passion so each of us can do the work we love, discover healthier and smarter energy sources, and find ways to share with those who are truly in need. We can set the intention and take appropriate action steps to support our families, the global community, and ourselves in the highest and best ways. It's a good time to ask, "What did I come to earth to do?"

My thoughts and feelings about money and abundance have changed dramatically over the years. I vividly remember having chest pains several times a month when I focused on lack of money—always on the days I paid the bills. I have had such a shift in thinking that I now joyfully write the checks each month as I send them off to pay utilities, insurance, and even the IRS. It is with a real sense of gratitude that I write a check to the electric company, because I have electricity that flows freely each time I turn on a switch. And they let me have it even before I pay for it! I'm thankful that I have the money to write the check and grateful for my talents and abilities to earn money.

My shift in thinking began in the late 1980s when I discovered a wonderful book, *Creating Money*, by Sanaya Roman and Duane Packer. It was instrumental in planting the seeds that have blossomed into my abundance garden. The contents of their book enabled me to examine why I had such negative and fearful thoughts about money and lack. In one particular exercise, the authors suggested to readers that they recall their earliest negative experience surrounding money.

A very poignant and old memory came to me quite readily. I recalled a time when I was five years old and was having great fun at a bingo game with my grandparents. I remembered squealing "Bingo!" and being absolutely thrilled when $7.50 was presented to me—the winner! In the early 1950s that was a *lot* of money, and at my age, I felt like a millionaire. People around me joined in my excitement and I was feeling so rich! Moments later, my grandmother asked me to look under the table for a bingo chip she had dropped. After retrieving it for her, I looked on the table and my money was gone. I remember feeling like my heart had dropped to my feet. I looked at my grandmother and asked what happened to the money. She replied, "I took it. I bought the bingo cards—it's my money. You're just a child." I started to cry and was told to "contain myself" and not to make a fuss.

That experience was pivotal in creating the belief that I was undeserving of money. I learned to repress my feelings. I came to believe I couldn't be trusted to handle money. I learned that people I loved sometimes did things that I couldn't understand.

I now realize that my grandmother experienced enormous fear and lack during the Great Depression and that living on a small pension made her scrape for each penny she could find. I now know that I am deserving of all good. After many years of silence, I now (almost always) express my feelings with compassion and honesty as they rise within me. I have learned so much about money and I continue to seek becoming more financially savvy. And I have learned the power of forgiveness.

If you are troubled by debt, or think money is "the root of all evil" (note: the Bible says that the *love* of money is the root of all evil, not money itself) or have blocks to believing you can have and spend money wisely, you may want to track the origin of those limiting beliefs. It can really help in clearing a way for spending and receiving money mindfully.

Forgiveness may be involved in this process of healing your negative beliefs about money or deprivation. Some people believe that credit card debt decreases as our level of forgiveness (of ourselves and others) increases. Could there be a connection between forgiveness and debt in your life? Committing to learning more about the nature of money and becoming familiar with financial planning strategies helps too.

Suze Orman, internationally acclaimed financial expert, has compiled numerous books and CDs filled with practical financial advice. One of my favorite tips from Suze is to save every bit of change you receive when paying with cash. For example, if you buy something for $9.50, pay with a $10 bill and save the coins. At the end of the day, put the change in a jar. At the end of the month or year, use that money to pay down debt or to invest. You'll be amazed at the amount you can collect in this effortless way.

The inspirational work of Esther and Jerry Hicks through Abraham-Hicks Publications (see bibliography) has been quite instrumental in my own shift of thinking about money and abundance. The idea of matching my "vibration" to what I want to attract is something I play with every day. For years, my attraction point would be one of lack and un-deservedness. And since that's what I thought, guess what I got? More of the same! As I have allowed myself to even think that it's okay for me to have more money, more money keeps coming my way. The more money I have, the more I can give.

I was raised to judge people with money—and it wasn't a flattering judgment. So it makes sense that I never wanted to be rich. Thankfully, I now focus on people with money who make a grand difference in this world. I want my money to make a difference. I want to **s**pend money with joy and wisdom. Do you?

It may be time to shift our collective thoughts from debt, lack, fear, and perceived deprivation to affluence, plentitude, and financial fulfillment. We can each take responsibility for creating our own financial stimulus plan. Stimulus is defined as "a thing that arouses activity or energy in someone or something." A stimulating thought gets us charged up and lets the energy zap out of us in a powerful, positive way. It erases the "poor me" (been there) and adds a "Yes we can" attitude to our financial lives.

What we focus on expands, so choose your thoughts with care. Give generously and joyfully. Receive graciously. Take charge of your spending habits by creating and implementing your own financial stimulus plan. Here are ten steps designed to expand, stimulate, and uplift your financial wellness plan.

Ten Steps to Creating Your Financial Wellness Stimulus Plan

1. The first step in creating a financial wellness stimulus plan is to write on a piece of paper, "I'm in! I am mindfully developing a sound plan for my money!" You switch the power button on when you put your plans in writing.

2. Next, take a deep breath and gather some facts. List how much you have in your checking and savings accounts. (Just in case you didn't do this after reading this tip in Chapter 11.) Take another deep breath and write down your retirement account balances. Speaking of breath, here is a powerful breathing method that can redirect your stressful thinking into a more relaxed state: Stop now and take a deep, full breath through your nose and hold it four seconds. Then gently and slowly exhale twice as long as your inhale. Repeat when necessary and observe the calming shift.

3. Do you have credit card debt? If you do, take a ledger sheet and write the account name, amount owed and the amount of finance charge for each account. Arrange this list from the highest APR to the lowest. (APR stands for annual percentage rate—the finance charge expressed as an annual rate, it's listed on your bill.) Pay off the highest rate first, while making timely payments on the others. Create a monthly plan and set payoff dates—even if the dates are far away. If you are unable to make these payments, call each company and make a plan to pay what you can. Consider

saving all your change and use it to help pay down credit card debt.

4. Write down everything you spend in one month. Save every receipt from today through the next 30 days and include cash items with no receipt like tips, pitching in on parking, or lunch expenses. Be meticulous. Knowing this number is actually empowering and most people (like me years ago) do everything to pretend they don't really need to know it. KNOW IT! What is the actual amount of money you spend in one month? This number is vital to your financial wellness stimulus plan. Keeping your head in the sand just gets your skin dry and your eyes itchy.

5. Write down all income sources and say "thank you" for every single dollar on that list. If you have lost your job or your hours have been cut, write down anything that comes your way—concentrate on what you have rather than the lack. And keep saying "thank you" to God for what you have.

6. Consider diversifying your income sources and developing a stream of residual income. This has resulted in a positive shift for me in the past several years and is the way I have replaced the 2008 hit to my retirement accounts.

7. Take all of this information and write down three action steps that can move you toward more financial abundance and stability.

8. If you have more than enough, consider sharing. Food banks would love your support, charities are open to volunteers as well as your checks, and family members in need might appreciate a gift card good at their local grocery store.

9. Observe your spending. Do you really, really *need* what you are about to buy? Put the money you were thinking of spending on that unnecessary item in your emergency fund.

(Okay, I'm still working on an emergency fund as part of the plan, but if you can pull it off, go for it! I am finding more success with residual income streams instead.)

10. Focus on what you want and what you have. It's often easy to get caught up in lack and worry. Remember, worrying is like praying for something you *don't* want. Believe, or borrow my belief, that you are always being cared for, and you will get through to the other side.

13

Cultivate Forgiveness

○ ○

You may never change the person who has wronged you, but in the course of loving an enemy, the life that is transformed is your own.

—*Mary Morrissey*

Cultivating forgiveness is a powerful way to plant the seeds for a more peaceful mind, body, and spirit. The most important thing I've learned about forgiveness is that it is not for the other person; it's for me.

I was given a great opportunity to learn about forgiveness in the early 1980s when I entered the hospital for a simple surgical procedure and the doctor accidentally severed an artery. After life-saving surgery, I was left with an unsightly scar and experienced many months of deep sadness and depression associated with this new body image. It finally occurred to me that I might need to forgive the doctor for the surgical mistake in order for me to heal my mind, body, and spirit.

I eventually went to see a very caring priest to discuss my feelings. I remember asking him if I had to forgive the doctor for the trauma he had caused. He quietly answered, "Yes, but not today. You'll forgive him when you are ready." His wise counsel enabled me to leave feeling empowered to choose when I wanted to forgive and not feel forced into it. I actually think that I forgave the doctor as the church doors closed behind me. The deeply profound sadness began to drift away and I realized that I was the one to reap the benefits from the healing powers of forgiveness. I believe my heart longed for the blessing of forgiveness more than it valued the pain that had been trapped inside it.

The act of forgiving doesn't make the other person's actions right or acceptable. When you choose to forgive, you set *yourself* free. Forgiveness frees you from the painful bond created between you and the other person through the actions or words that caused the wound in the relationship. Sometimes I am aware enough to ask myself the question, "Do I want to heal it or hang on to it?" I usually choose the healing route. I am now able to call the person to mind and mentally say, "Thank you FOR GIVING me the opportunity to learn and grow and heal a part of me that was seeking to be healed." Sometimes I don't get it all out of me on the first try—so I say it and pray it again when necessary. Like cultivating the soil by pulling out the unwanted weeds, I dig deeper to prepare a more receptive place for the healing seeds to sprout and flourish.

Neal Donald Walsch wrote a delightfully touching children's book that I recommend to adults. My friend Karen read his book *The Little Soul and the Sun: A Children's Parable Adapted from Conversations With God* to me over the phone when I was experiencing a particularly painful passage in my life. Part of the story shares the idea that we somehow make a kind of "soul-agreement" with people who come into our lives to teach us lessons that open our hearts wider. The Little Soul wanted to learn about forgiveness, so of course, he needed to have someone to forgive. A precious little girl soul stepped up and agreed to enter the world with him, but only if he agreed to remember who she really, really was. This tender parable broadened my thinking about forgiveness and soothed my own soul in the process.

Consider learning about the powerful Hawaiian practice of reconciliation and forgiveness called Ho'oponopono, mentioned in Chapter 9. The simple, peaceful, and poignant lines are: Dear God (Or whatever you call the Divine) I am sorry. Please forgive me. I love you. And I thank you. If you want to view a tenderly beautiful seven minute meditation, type in "Ho'oponopono Meditation Mantra and Prayer" in the YouTube search engine.

It has been said that un-forgiveness is like drinking poison and expecting the other person to die. Sometimes when I become aware of any poison I am carrying within, I have found it helpful to write a letter of forgiveness, where I pour out everything I think and feel about the situation. Sometimes it may be important to send the letter, but most often I have chosen to burn the letter after quiet words of prayer, with an intention of release and healing for all involved. (I do appreciate having a fireplace.) If you write a letter that you think needs to be sent, I recommend holding on to it for a few days first, just to be sure that is the action you really want to take. If you are sending it to get a certain response from the other person, I'd suggest mailing the letter back to yourself instead. I usually find I have already said what needed to be said to the person, or realize the other person would be unable to really hear what I had to say, so simply writing the letter provided me the opportunity to scrape out the last of the poison that was contaminating the garden of my own heart. I have also discovered times when I needed to write a letter of forgiveness to myself. When I write these letters, I have a sense of my most loving self holding the pen. A sense of relief usually follows the signature.

Do you know someone you might want to forgive? You will, when you are ready.

Ways to Cultivate Forgiveness

1. Take a few deep breaths and let the face or name of a person you want to forgive come into your mind.

2. Decide if you are ready to fully forgive this person now or if you just want to start the process. You don't have to do it all today. Notice that, and make your decision.

3. If you are unable to forgive the person now, ask yourself what you might need to give up in order to do so. It might be giving up the need to be right. Sometimes it's the idea that feeling like a victim somehow provides a sense of protection. Sometimes you truly are a victim and soon you may choose to step away from that role and think of yourself as a survivor. Sometimes it just seems like forgiveness requires giving up something (usually a belief) you've held onto for so long that it would feel strange to release it.

4. Consider writing a letter and getting out all your uncensored thoughts and feelings. Don't feel the need to be sweet or kind here, blast it out on that paper! You may want to choose to share this with a trusted friend so you can be heard and not judged. If so, ask them to listen but not to comment. You may choose to read your letter to God. You may choose to scream it to God. I DO NOT suggest sending this letter or reading it to the person who committed the offense. Don't even be tempted. This isn't for them; it's for you—all for you. Then burn or shred the letter as you see fit.

5. Bring this person to your mind again and say, "I forgive you," but only when you are ready. You may even ask God to be at your side as you gather the courage to take this step. Consider using the words found in the powerful Hawaiian practice of reconciliation and forgiveness called Ho'oponopono: Dear God (Or whatever you call the Divine) I am sorry. Please forgive me. I love you. And I thank you. You may need to repeat this last step as many times as necessary until finally, you feel the tremendous blessing that seeps into the places that once hurt so deeply.

14

Practice Peace

○ ○

Let there be peace on earth and let it begin with me.
—Jill Jackson and Sy Miller

Peace begins at home, home within the center of each of us. Our peaceful state of mind can then be extended to our family, friends, community, and the world. It can even be extended to people who don't believe as we do. If we each take steps to promote this harmony, we could eventually see peace reach epidemic proportions.

It is often easy to condemn groups of people who are at war with each other. We may shake our heads wondering why "they" can't live in peace. But are we living in peace? Are we at peace with ourselves? People creating terror hold a grudge against people who do not think like they do. Do we harbor grudges against family, former partners, coworkers, or neighbors? I believe if each of us takes the steps necessary to truly practice peace "at home," within our bodies and souls, then it will be easier to sustain a peace consciousness throughout our entire planet.

Nelson Mandela and François Pienaar offered the world a profound example of peace as they combined efforts that greatly enhanced the healing of the people in South Africa post-apartheid. The unique relationship that developed between this unlikely duo is the theme of the 2009 film *Invictus*. President Mandela supported rugby captain François Pienaar and the almost all-white rugby team as they focused united efforts that resulted in the 1995 World Cup victory for South

Africa. It seems they weren't just practicing rugby; they were also practicing peace.

I find I must make a conscious and repeated effort to keep out the fearful energy that seems so prominent both nationally and across the globe. On one of my business trips post-September 11, I noticed a creeping tension in my neck as the voice over the loudspeaker repeatedly barked that I could not take liquids in my carry-on luggage. As I observed people removing their shoes and putting their belongings in the gray plastic bins to be x-rayed, I wondered how someone might view this scene if he or she had just awakened from a ten-year coma. How long would it take for the person to go from viewing this scene as a crazy joke to developing a pain in *her* neck? Is it possible to transform this fear-filled thinking back into a focus on peace? Yes, I believe it is, and I will spend the rest of my life working toward that goal.

You can too. Every day, you can choose to create peace within your own heart. When listening to the radio or watching the evening news, you can take deep breaths and a moment to pray for peace. You might even choose to create a ritual of peace-thinking in your daily life. For example, every time you stop at a red light, it could be a signal to *think peace* and *be peace*. I love the peace bumper stickers I see when I'm driving too. And I giggle out loud every time I see the one that says, "Envision Whirled Peas"!

I invite you to join me in mindfully taking time to pray for peace, within ourselves first and then throughout the world. Whether you walk through the doorway of your own home or through the metal doorway in airport security, dare to be the carrier of peace.

If fear has created elaborate security systems at airports, why not use this as an opportunity rather than consider it a nuisance? And why couldn't there be elaborate places to pray and meditate right next to the security checkpoints? Even a simple place would do. I have visions of airports creating small meditation or prayer spots that people can enjoy while they are putting their shoes back on their feet. Most airports have small chapels hidden out of sight. Why not relocate them and plop them in plain (and plane) sight? Why not create peace arches as gateways through the metal detectors? This would be an excellent place to pray for the people we call "terrorists," and, even more crucial, to pray that we might live our lives without the slightest thought of any kind of violence or intimidation against others.

There are bright spots as individuals and organizations daily create peace in big and small ways. I shed a few tears when I read a poster (sponsored by Raventalk) on the underground train while riding from one concourse to another in the Denver airport. It contained the following quote by Longfellow: "If we could read the secret history of our enemies, we would find in each personal story enough suffering and sorrow there to disarm all hostilities."

It was on that same trip to Denver in 2006 that I had the privilege of teaching Nia to children who were refugees from the African countries of Somalia, Uganda, Sierra Leone, Mauritania, Rwanda, and the Democratic Republic of the Congo. (You will read more about Nia in the next chapter.) My daughter and her colleagues had planned and facilitated the first-ever Peace Pals Leadership Summit for these children at Mt. Evans Outdoor Education Laboratory in Evergreen, Colorado. In this newly formed Peace Pal program, children ages 6 – 17 were taught three basic concepts: don't bully others, include others who feel left out, and tell adults when someone is being bullied.

The focus for the Nia class was peace. I read the quote to the children that I have often shared in my adult classes:

"Peace. It does not mean to be in a place where there is no noise, trouble, or hard work. It means to be in the midst of those things and still be calm in your heart."

This quote from an unknown source reminds me to seek the peace within, even amidst the chaos. The children seemed drawn to this gentle message. As they danced (some of the children had never been seen moving their bodies with any kind of free expression before this class), they used their voices to join me in shouts of "yes!" and "no!" and blocked and wriggled and wiggled and twirled. They floated their hands in front of their hearts and gestured to each other as they gleefully sang from the chorus of one of the songs, "You're beautiful forever!"

At the end of the class, we gathered in a circle and I asked the children to close their eyes, cover their hearts with their hands, and call to mind someone or some place that they wanted to send peace to at that moment. One little girl softly uttered, "Africa!" The sacred circle of children settled into silence with faces exuding hope, trust, love, and peace. Right then, I wanted to take them all home with me for a visit. But then I remembered the giggles and the coughing and the silly bodily sounds and the snoring that kept me up the night before (this was, after all, a camping experience) and I was quickly brought back to reality. But I also sealed into my cells—from the beauty of these children and the Rocky Mountains—the profound feeling and reality of that peace-filled moment.

And speaking of sealing this peace into our cells, don't think it can't be done. Jill Bolte Taylor, Ph. D., the neuroanatomist I mentioned in Chapter 4, wrote this after documenting her own experience of recovering from a rare form of stroke: "I believe the more time we spend running our deep inner peace circuitry, then the more peace we will project into the world, and ultimately the more peace we will have on the planet."

When we practice peace in all parts of our daily life, we could actually begin to upset the condition of conflict and turmoil in the world. Practice peace. Think peace. Be peace. Touch peace. It's communicable.

Twelve Suggestions for Practicing Peace

1. Bring to mind a part of your life that would benefit from an infusion of peace. Ask yourself if you are ready and willing to take steps to create more peace around this situation. Ask for peace to enter.

2. Meet conflict with awareness, directness, compassion, and a desire to seek a solution. Keep in mind that conflict isn't bad, it's choosing verbal or physical violence to attempt to resolve the conflict that is so harmful. Conflict can lead to a greater understanding between two people or two nations—or ten nations. Remember Longfellow's quote: "If we could read the secret history of our enemies, we would find in each

personal story enough suffering and sorrow there to disarm all hostilities."

3. Refuse to participate in violent thinking or actions. Be aware of thoughts directed toward yourself or others that may be harmful. Refuse to watch violent films or listen to music with lyrics that degrade, or reflect violent speech or actions.

4. When you feel angry or upset, acknowledge your feelings before attempting to release them. Sometimes anger comes up when we don't like how we are being treated. Anger can be a helpful signal that alerts you to make choices to keep you safe. Be lovingly aware that frequent states of agitation or anger take you farther away from peace.

5. Do not stuff these feelings inside or ignore them, but wisely choose to observe them rather than act out in anger. You may need to do something physical (running, riding a bike, gardening, chopping wood) to get the anger up, out, and through you. After you have physically expelled the anger, you may want to listen to calming music, take a walk in nature, or funnel your energy into a project that creates a space for expanded peace.

6. Learn more about nonviolent communication, often referred to as compassionate communication, through the work of Marshall Rosenberg. (See bibliography.) The Center for Nonviolent Communication www.cnvc.org defines nonviolence as "the natural state of compassion when no violence is present in the heart."

7. When you are with a family member, neighbor, co-worker, or anyone who presses your buttons, pause and take a deep breath. (It's best to do this deep breathing thing subtly.) Make a choice to respond rather than react. You may simply say something like, "Really? That's interesting." Then, put imaginary duct tape over your buttons and refuse to

react when someone attempts to press them. Remember, someone might be pressing your buttons but they didn't install them.

8. Respect yourself and others by choosing not to use any profanity or comments that degrade or puts someone down. This includes your own self-talk.

9. Speak out for those who are disrespected. Choose words that do not blame or judge. You may choose to be an advocate for people who have been abused, disregarded, degraded, or have experienced unthinkable acts of violence. Nicholas D. Kristof and Sheryl WuDunn, winners of the Pulitzer Prize and the authors of *Half the Sky: Turning Oppression into Opportunity for Women Worldwide,* offer an extensive list of groups who provide support for the oppressed. Check out the list in their Appendix if you feel stirred to action.

10. Be open to understanding ideas and people you have previously opposed. Dare to discover where you can find common ground. Exploring what both sides can be *for* rather than *against* is always a good place to start. The other person doesn't need to be wrong to make you right.

11. Dare to think about just one significant way you can work more effectively with the people in your workplace, school, or community. Then take action to put that idea into place. Observe how peacefully working together creates stronger individuals and communities. A simple pledge to not participate in gossip is a good starting place.

12. Smile more often, at yourself and others. Smiles, and peace, are communicable

15

Discover the Joys of Movement

○ ○
Jump.

—*Joseph Campbell*

Years ago I noticed how certain words with similar meanings prompted different reactions. I stopped saying "exercise" when I discovered that my next thought was "No pain, no gain." That didn't sound like much fun for me, so I began substituting the word "movement" for "exercise." My clients smiled and their bodies relaxed when I would suggest they find a form of *movement* that would be just right for them.

While in my mid-forties, I could not always find a tennis or racquetball partner and sometimes felt bored lifting weights or riding a cycle that went nowhere. I had taken jazz dance classes for years but my work schedule often conflicted with the class schedule. During this time I discovered a holistic form of movement called Nia. Nia is a transformational fusion fitness and lifestyle practice that blends selected movements from the martial arts, the dance arts, and the healing arts. Nia uses *The Body's Way* to achieve physical, mental, emotional, and spiritual health and well-being. Anyone can enjoy Nia because it encourages all participants to listen to the wisdom of their bodies. It brings out the inner dancer in everyone—especially in people who were told in their childhood (or adulthood) that they couldn't dance or were too clumsy. All sizes, shapes, and ages can joyfully participate. If you are in a wheelchair or have a limited range of motion, you can enjoy the arm movements, music, sensations, sounds, and images created through Nia routines.

I discovered a passion for Nia that continues to inspire me to want to care for and nourish all aspects of my being. I am a certified black belt Nia instructor and have been teaching since 1999. I delight in being a dancing grandmother! And I must share this—I got a kick out of turning 60 in 2009 and love being able to get down and get back up again with ease! Nia has opened the doorway to profound joy, healing, passion, and wholeness in my life and in the lives of Nia students across the globe.

You can learn more by taking a Nia class or by reading *The Nia Technique—The High-Powered Energizing Workout That Gives You a New Body and a New Life* by Nia co-creators Debbie Rosas and Carlos AyaRosas. If you visit the Web site www.NiaNow.com you will find listings for classes all over the world.

Dance and martial arts don't excite you? Simply walking each day can bring a sense of calm and provide cardiovascular benefits. If you move through your day via wheelchair or a Segway, taking time to get outside and connect your wheels to the earth can heighten your awareness as you take in all that surrounds you. If you like cycling or in-line skating, you can do that with attention to what's flying by you. Whether you are walking, rolling, or jogging you can feel the wind on your face and through your hair. Delight in your senses. Smell the moment, see what you are traveling in and around, touch a flower or a rock or tree. Twenty to 30 minutes of movement each day freshens the mind and gently massages the heart in many ways. If you walk or roll everywhere you go, make time to do a part of it with a real intention of being fully in your body; an intention and recognition of "being here now" rather than on your way someplace else.

If health concerns seriously limit your ability to move, I offer a pearl of wisdom that my mother's hospice counselor, Randi, suggested to her. Just a few days before my mother passed away, she confided in Randi that she realized she would never dance again. This wise and compassionate counselor took my mother's hand and said, "Helen, close your eyes, and let's dance together right now." The mind is magnificent, and my mother smiled as she enjoyed visions of dancing one last time. Let your imagination guide you to enjoyable places now. Don't wait.

It's important to note that some people don't have the problem of finding a movement form that suits them—they have found something and over-do it to the detriment of their body/mind. And in this arena of health concerns, if you or someone you love deals with disordered eating and over-exercising, Peach Friedman's captivating book, *Diary of an Exercise Addict*, provides inspiration and support for healing.

And so, I advocate closing your eyes for a moment and thinking of a form of movement that creates joyful feelings and suits *your* wellness path. This joyful activity is the one to start with if you're seeking a way to add more movement to your life. After selecting your first option, you might want to see if this movement involves strength, flexibility, and a cardiovascular benefit. (Nia provides all of these, by the way.) If not, the next step would be to consider adding another type of movement that includes these elements. Let this form of movement stir your passion and your pleasure.

Suggestions for Implementing the Ideas in This Chapter

1. Think of a form of movement that creates joyful feelings and suits *your* wellness path. Nia, yoga, tennis, jogging, hiking, Pilates, golf, dancing, biking, aerobics, tai chi, softball, skiing, rock climbing, swimming, walking, skating—these are just some of the choices you have.

2. Does this movement involve strength, flexibility, and a cardiovascular benefit? If not, the next step would be to consider adding another type of movement that includes these elements.

3. Consider working out with a buddy. This is a great way to motivate and support both of you in creating time to discover the many joys of movement.

4. Walking is a wonderful way to provide cardio-vascular benefits. Have fun stretching before and after you walk

and you've added flexibility into your plan. If you have a gym membership, add weights and "play" with how it feels to strengthen your body. An alternative is to buy weights (second-hand stores always seem to have this type of equipment around) and check with a personal trainer or find a good book from the library to guide you. Less is more in this arena, as you never want to strain your muscles. It's important to skip a day to allow your muscle fibers to rebuild properly. So if you do an upper body workout one day, focus on lower body the next.

5. Set the intention to participate in healthy movement activities every two days. Seek pleasure in your choices, be playful, and don't overdo.

16

Revel in Relaxation

○ ○
Relax and let the river flow . . . let your life lead you where you need to go!

—Jana Stanfield and Greg Tamblyn

Relaxation—don't you just love the sound of that word? I substituted the word "relaxation" for "stress management" a while ago because it seemed to jump right into the center of where I wanted to be—relaxed! How do you relax? When do you relax? Do you let others around you know when you are creating this relaxation time for yourself?

If I had one thing to do over, it would be to schedule more time to take care of *me*. I've finally learned (now that I am a grandmother) I am much better able to care for others when I have cared for myself first. Should you be accused of being selfish, I'd suggest saying, "No, I'm being self-*full*!" If this concept challenges your way of thinking, you might recall the image of a flight attendant instructing parents to secure their own masks before assisting their small children.

Our youngest child, Molly, was eight years old when I decided I would lock the bathroom door, light candles, play soft music, and ease into a tub of soothing bubbles—alone. Even though I went around the house to see if anyone needed anything before I retreated to the bathroom and announced I would be unavailable for the next 30 minutes, that first time was a shock to the family. Five minutes later, Molly was knocking on the door. Soon our son Zack "really needed" me and I found my relaxation efforts had turned into a bad comedy skit. So, I recognize this step might take some practice for everyone, but just keep making the time and insisting upon it. You are worth it and people around you will also reap the rewards.

If you intentionally create a reasonable bedtime and plug in just a bit of extra time in the morning, you have the opportunity to start your day with ease. If you awaken to a baby's cry, children squealing, or if you are the caregiver of another family member, it may be all you can do to take a deep breath before bolting out of bed. When possible, take a few gentle breaths before allowing your feet to gently step into your day.

We all relax in different ways. You can listen to music, read, watch movies, walk, garden, feed the birds, sew, work in the garage, or create art. Pick *your* way and plug it into your daily life whenever possible. Relaxation is a wonderful way to enhance your wellness wisdom.

Whether you live alone or with others, it is important to take time to replenish yourself as you revel in relaxation. Do you need ideas to help extract yourself from the stresses of daily life to even *get* to the possibility of reveling in relaxation? Here are ten tips to support you in moving out of stress mode and into the pleasures of relaxation. Pick one or two to add to your wellness practices now and add others gently in the times that follow.

Ten Tips to Reduce Stress and Enhance Relaxation

1. Awaken with ease. Does your alarm clock jolt you from the serenity of sleep? Harsh buzzing noises can ignite the fight or flight response, secreting cortisol into your bloodstream—not a good way to start your day. Cortisol is a chemical often referred to as the "stress hormone" since it is involved in the response to stress. It increases blood pressure, raises blood sugar levels, and has an immunosuppressive action. One way to reduce stress from the moment you wake up is to choose a pleasing alarm clock. There are many alarm options these days, including clocks that can awaken you with music, sunrise simulators, nature sounds, aromatherapy, or my new favorite, a Zen-like gong. On the days when I need to rise at a specific time, I now awaken to a digitally reproduced

recording of a Tibetan gong bowl. It's delightful! I was so excited to hear it that for the first week I kept waking up long before it was set to go off. For me, this peaceful sound generates a sacred feeling to the start of the day. What works best for you?

2. Meditate and/or pray. Plugging in five minutes of quiet meditation or prayer right after you awaken has the ability to profoundly affect the direction of your day. Fifteen minutes is even better, but starting with five minutes will create amazing results. You can do this before getting out of bed or find a place where you can sit quietly without being disturbed. If other family members require your attention at this time of day, set aside some time during the day when you can just pause. It's cheaper than a latte and can be deeply satisfying. (Or you can totally enjoy your morning coffee as a meditation dessert!)

3. Eat a nourishing breakfast. It's so easy to grab the first "meal" of the day on the run or even wait until mid-morning to gulp down a muffin while you stand by the kitchen sink or sit in front of your computer. There's a reason breakfast is known to be the most important meal of the day. It breaks the "fast" from dinner and is absolutely crucial in providing essential nutrients for your day. If you don't eat breakfast, that cortisol kicks in and your body thinks it's starving. Then, when you do eat at lunch time, your stomach still isn't ready to digest your food because the cortisol is supporting your stressful fight or flight mode by preparing the body to be chased by a bear (or a grumpy boss). So, your lunch just hangs out in your stomach for an extra amount of time and eventually creates extra pounds around your middle, causing more stress. We don't let our car get to empty before we re-fuel. It's equally important to keep our body's fuel supply steady for our best running condition and to reduce stress.

4. Take high quality supplements. Supporting our cells with vitamins and minerals is crucial these days. The American Medical Association (AMA), previously saying little about the need for vitamins, now encourages daily vitamin supplementation. (Learn more from the 2002 *Journal of the American Medical Association* resource listed in the bibliography.) When we nourish our cells at the most basic level, we give our bodies the opportunity to thrive, increase our ability to handle the daily stressors of life, help to prevent degenerative disease, and control damage produced by free radicals.

5. Be in the present. I cover this topic in Chapter 29, but if you don't get to it today, here's the gem: the present really is a gift you give yourself. When we let the concerns of the past or fears of the future enter into this precious second, we create stress. Stop. Breathe in. Breathe out. Be.

6. Provide service. When we provide service to others, we also support ourselves. Being of service is a real stress-buster if we are doing things we love, in a passionate way and without expectation of return. I have a little Post-it note on my computer that says, "What do you have for me to do today God? How can I be of service?" It is a guide for each conversation and each task I assume. Engaging in providing service doesn't mean I "help" people, because that would put me on a higher plane and others below me. Rather, I offer service from a realization of oneness, as a fellow human traveler offering the best of who I am at this moment. It doesn't mean giving unsolicited advice or telling people how they can make their life better when they didn't ask you. It may simply mean listening—being fully present—to what someone is saying. Service may mean sharing your music, art, or other talents with others. It may mean volunteering or working in a soup kitchen. It may mean working as a grocery clerk and offering a kind word to someone whose nasty behavior indicates he is having a really bad day. (I have

heard that the amount of pain a person inflicts on others is directly proportional to the amount of pain that person feels within himself.) It may mean being all that you are, in whatever work you do, so that you can make a difference in this world. Provide service, release stress!

7. Seek pleasure. Be a pleasure-seeking arrow, always on the lookout for a great, joyful target. Awaken with pleasure, work with pleasure, love with pleasure, pray with pleasure, provide service with pleasure, work out with pleasure, eat with pleasure, breathe with pleasure. Or, you could concentrate on searching for things that aggravate you or cause tension and stress. It's your choice.

8. Breathe. Taking three breaths before you begin to eat is quite a quick entry into a more relaxed state. It relaxes the digestive system, so you can better receive the food you are feeding your body. Are you feeling tense when stuck in traffic? Come back home to your breath. Breathing in—and breathing out. Getting ready for an important meeting or potentially challenging conversation? Breathe. Our breath is such a treasure if we choose to simply call upon it with mindfulness and awareness.

9. Tell the people you love that you love them. We can do this in person, on the phone, in e-mail, on Facebook, or by sending a silent message to a special heart. Be sure to be unattached to any expectation of reciprocation, as that can add stress rather than dispel it. Love is a vital nutrient that can gently melt away the stressors that sometimes surround us. Don't forget to send some loving messages to yourself too. And out of the mouths of babes: "You really shouldn't say 'I love you' unless you mean it. But if you mean it, you should say it a lot. People forget." (Jessica, age 8)

10. Be grateful. Calling attention to gratitude is a magical tool for reveling in relaxation. When we call to mind the people and things we are grateful for, we may discover that the

dramas of life are temporarily placed aside, the loneliness is put on hold, the fear dissipates, and our focus rests on extraordinarily simple pleasures. As you'll read in Chapter 31, nighttime is a great time to bless the day with thoughts of gratitude. Or don't wait until bedtime; feel free to take a moment and think of just one thing you are grateful for right now.

17

Reframe Worrying

Never trouble trouble till trouble troubles you!
—Unknown but spoken most often by my dear friend,
Phyllis Fontana

Are you really good at worrying? Do you believe that it makes you a better person (partner, mother, father, daughter, son, friend) if you worry about someone? Do you think your level of worry has a direct correlation to keeping a loved one safe? Do you think having a high level of worry proves your love for someone? If so, here's a new view to consider: *worrying does not protect your loved ones and it takes a lot of energy away from your daily activities.* Might there be a better use for your time and energy?

I believe women are particularly good at worrying. (And clearly, I have known some really good worriers who are men.) I have often wondered if a mother's genetic coding convinces her that worrying about her children will earn her the mother-of-the-year award. Well, I gave up worrying when my son, Zack, turned 16 and began driving. That's when I realized that worrying had no correlation with his safety. There just wasn't enough time or energy to focus all my thoughts in that negative way—so I switched to envisioning him safe and realized that if he wasn't, I would be able to handle it. I discovered that sometimes he was safe and sometimes he wasn't. I learned I really couldn't control what was happening in his life; I could only attempt to control how I thought about it in my life. Zack is now in his thirties and I notice that "concern" often creeps into my thinking, but rarely "worry." Sometimes he hasn't been safe—and I've survived. Fortunately, so has he.

This concept of not worrying has come in handy as both of my adult children continue on unique career paths that sometimes take them far from home. My daughter, Molly, earned a master's degree in International Disaster Psychology and spent her internship working with an organization for unaccompanied children in Bosnia. She has been on peace trips to Northern Ireland and the Balkans, and has studied in Senegal and France. Zack tours the country sharing his awesome music and is often on the road. Our time together, when we get it, is precious.

It is the norm to admonish to our children, "Be careful!" At some point, I remember consciously feeling better when I sent them off with a feeling of love rather than fear. I remember saying to my kids, as they left the house as teens, "Have a great time! I'll see you when you get home." The implication was that I trusted them to return safely rather than feared for their safety.

Kahlil Gibran wrote, "Your children are not your children. They are the sons and daughters of Life's longing for itself . . . You are the bows from which your children as living arrows are sent forth." It is crucial for parents to hold the bow strong and steady and equally important to release the arrows from that bow so they fly forward on their own path.

A few years ago, Molly accepted a position working as a counselor for the United Nations in Burundi, a country located south of Rwanda in East Africa. She drove UN vehicles to work that were inspected for explosives before she entered the mission. She traveled by convoy and sometimes by helicopter to provide services for UN workers in remote areas. (I distinctly remember one phone conversation when Molly described watching the pilot load her stress management materials onto the helicopter, next to the ammunition.)

At this writing, she is a program manager for a non-government organization (NGO) located in Burundi. She offers support and training for people working with child soldiers and victims of human trafficking in several regions in East Africa and in Sri Lanka. Her arrow continues to fly.

People often ask me if I worry about her. "No," I reply, "I don't." If I did, I'm sure I would be sick, sad, and a total wreck. And of course I haven't perfected this not-worrying thing 100 percent of the time. I am far from perfect! There have been times with both Molly and Zack when I struggled to bring my thoughts back to seeing them safe, particularly when they were traveling and the communication lines were quiet. But it is clear to me, worrying is not the best use of my mind power.

And I must repeatedly and mindfully choose not to worry about Zack. He is an amazing singer-songwriter who travels in and out of cities and stays who-knows-where on any given occasion. I have deep respect for his unique spirit, as he creates an artist's path that is often forged "out of the box" of society's expectations of success. His music rocks my soul and just thinking of his heart and being brings tears to my eyes.

Our children were not put on his earth to please us or to follow a path that we choose for them. They get to create their passion. The best way I can support them is to honor who they are and hold them in a vision of health, light, safety, and love. My intention is to surround them with prayerful thoughts of safety, love, and well-being. I am filled with awe for their accomplishments. They are unique individuals with their own strengths. They are not an extension of me.

Are there adult children in your life who are forging their own way through this twenty-first century world? Do you spend precious time worrying about them? Would your time be better spent loving them, respecting them, envisioning them surrounded by light and safety? It's wise and supports everyone's journey of wellness to allow these individual arrows to find their own target.

Gay Hendricks suggests in his book, *The Big Leap*, that worrying is an addiction. Now that thought grabbed my attention! (So did the rest of his book.) The kicker is, we sometimes hit the jackpot (and feel rewarded) when something we worry about actually comes true. In Hendricks' words, "If you worry long enough about the stock market crashing, you'll eventually hit the jackpot, because from time to time it's always going to crash."

Worrying just isn't worth the energy drain, is it? The next time you feel worried, try replacing that thought with a prayer or a trusting image and see if it makes you feel less angst. For some, this might take a while to reprogram a very old pattern of thinking. But you will discover the reframing is worth the effort.

I once heard that worrying over the things we can't control is a waste of time because we can't control them. Worrying over the things we can control is a waste of time because we can control them. So, why worry?

What do you value more, peace of mind or worrying? Maybe Bobby McFarrin has the right idea in his old refrain, "Don't worry, be happy!"

Seven Steps to Support You in Implementing the Ideas in This Chapter

1. Write down the name of someone or a situation you are worried about right now.

2. How does it make you physically feel when you think about that person or situation?

3. Write down what you can do, if anything, to control the situation.

4. Write down what you can't control.

5. How would you feel if you gave up worrying?

6. Do you want to keep on worrying or mindfully choose other things to think about or do?

7. Create a prayer or affirming statement that supports you in switching your thinking away from worrying mode. (Check out the Affirmations at the end of this book for ideas.) Say a prayer or state your affirmation each time worry enters your thoughts. Envision your loved ones surrounded by safety and light.

18

Letting Go

Attachment to outcome . . . BIG problem!
—His Holiness the Dalai Lama

You need to know right up front, this topic is a big one—letting go. However, I have truly found life to be so much easier when I let go of trying to control the outcome of things, people, and events. It takes so much emotional energy to cling to things we think we can control. When we let go, we gain the time and energy to accomplish so much more in our daily lives. Have you found this to be true?

While we're on the topic of letting go, are you willing to let go of shame, blame, and guilt? I see no redeeming value in this trio of beliefs. Oh, if we could only remove the damage these fear-based concepts have caused children and adults. I am not saying that we should adopt a ruthless, egotistical, and unconscious mindset. We need our conscience to help us with right and wrong. But I believe we could heal ourselves, the world, and support the healing of others if we made our decisions, as Elisabeth Kübler-Ross advocated, based on *love* rather than *fear*.

It had once been my nature to cling ferociously to the belief that I was powerful enough to change the thinking of family members, friends, and even entire university committees. I am mighty powerful— but not in that way. I know that my true power comes from honestly and compassionately speaking my truth with integrity, kindness, and compassion and then letting go of the outcome. And it's especially important to let go of the outcome. Pain has always resulted when I got in there and tried to force that oversized round peg into a very small square hole.

Trusting (rather than hoping) that things will unfold with ease in a way that is best for all involved will help as you prepare to truly let go. You may want to consider replacing the word *hope* with the word *trust*. Hope often implies something we wish might happen in the future. Trust can be a more optimistic and affirming way toward creating a specific result. And sometimes, it's appropriate to really, really hope.

A real lesson in trusting and letting go came when my father was living his last few years of life with Alzheimer's disease. My dear, rational, calm, clear thinking dad would tell me stories of flying boxcars that took him to work (and back) and he would tell me that wherever he landed, his bed would be right there too! The first time he told me this, I felt like my heart was bleeding tears. I felt desperate to bring him back into my reality. "Dad," I softly pleaded, "You know that part of your brain that isn't always connecting quite right? Well, that's what's happening now and that story isn't really true." I thought I was controlling the situation quite nicely. What an illusion!

When I let go and realized that his reality was *his* reality and totally different from mine, I began to find peace. I let go—and met him where he was, not where I wanted him to be. On one of our last walks together, I said, "Dad, tell me more about the boxcar with wings." His face lit up as he described how this unique train took off and landed so smoothly and how much fun it was to ride it. Dad had been a railroad engineer so the added speed created by the airplane wings must have been quite a delight for him! And my delight came when I was able to let go and be *with* him right where he was. For a while after his death, I spent time wishing I had met him there sooner. Now I know I did the best I could at the time. I know he knows it too.

Anthropologist Ralph Blum said, "Relinquishing control is the ultimate challenge for the spiritual warrior." We have a choice to cling to thoughts and beliefs that keep us stuck, in pain or in the illusion of control—or, we can let go, and let God handle the details. It's your choice.

Five Ways to Practice Letting Go

1. Explore and observe where there may be blame, shame, or guilt lurking anywhere in your mind. When you are ready, make a decision to release those thoughts and feelings if they no longer serve you.

2. List one or two situations in your life you wish you could control but deep down, you know you really can't. Visualize what it would feel like if you gave up the need to control that situation. Decide when, or if, you would like to let go.

3. A mentor of mine advocates, "Stand up, tell the truth, and get out of the way!" The "getting out of the way" piece is often the most challenging. Practice this technique if you like. Notice whether or not you can really get out of the way and let go of the outcome.

4. Trust, rather than hope, things will unfold in the perfect way. Notice if trusting feels more powerful than hoping.

5. Bring to mind the "let go, let God" thought when you need some divine intervention.

19

Laugh Often

At the height of laughter, the universe is flung into a kaleidoscope of new possibilities.

—Jean Houston

When was the last time you had a good, hearty laugh? You might want to rent a funny movie or find a good book that is sure to make you giggle. The endorphins we release when we laugh may work faster than aspirin.

The list of health benefits of laughter is much more fun to read than the list of possible side effects for almost any medication. Laughter lowers blood pressure, boosts the immune system, stimulates both sides of the brain, protects the heart, elevates mood, decreases stress, and above all—it makes you feel good!

Medical professionals are increasingly aware of the positive effects laughter has on the body and in the mind. Dr. Madan Kataria, an enlightened physician from India, gave birth to what he calls "Laughter Yoga." In the midnineties, after writing a medical journal article entitled "Laughter is the Best Medicine," he was so convinced of the many medical benefits of laughter, that he developed this new style of yoga to bring laughter into and through the body. Known as the Guru of Giggling, Dr. Kataria is responsible for Laughter Yoga's popularity in over 6,000 laughter clubs and studios in more than 60 countries. The "Guru of Giggling": wouldn't you love to have that title on your business card?

A team of University of Maryland School of Medicine researchers, led by Dr. Michael Miller, conducted a study using laughter-provoking movies to assess the effect of emotions in relation to cardiovascular health. The results reported in 2005 indicate that laughter is linked to the healthy functioning of blood vessels. Dr. Miller comments, "The recommendation for a healthy heart may one day be exercise, eat right, and laugh a few times a day." What a great prescription!

Can you laugh at yourself? Some of us may have memories from our childhood when people taunted or teased us with malicious laughter. This may have resulted in us not being able to laugh at our own follies. Consider being lighter. The laughter we generate can be so healing, as long as it isn't directed at someone in the form of ridicule.

Laughter is contagious too, and much more fun to catch than a virus. If you find you don't have much to laugh about, you may want to examine your daily choices. You and only you can make the change to bring more laughter into your life. Laughter can truly be our best medicine.

Three Suggestions for Implementing the Ideas in This Chapter

1. Laugh often.

2. Laugh some more. Funny films are helpful!

3. If it feels good, laugh some more.

20

Embrace Intimacy

○ ○

Love and intimacy are at a root [sic] of what makes us sick and what makes us well, what causes sadness and what brings happiness, what make us suffer and what leads to healing.

—Dean Ornish, M.D.

You may have heard that if you say the word "intimacy" slowly, you might hear the words "in-to-me-see." Some find it challenging to let anyone see right into them, to feel so vulnerable. At times it may seem safer to build a protective wall around your heart to form a shield from the pain of potential loss or rejection. That kind of wall only serves to amplify our human longing for love and closeness. Now that's pain.

Mary Morrissey, writing in *No Less Than Greatness—Finding Perfect Love in Imperfect Relationships*, provides insights for tender hearts in her words, "It's in the midst of the pain—those times when the tendency is to hold back—that we have the greatest opportunity for perfect loving."

If your heart has been wounded or broken, you may want to break your heart one more time—break it wide open. Crack it so wide that it's open to all the good that healing can bring. In her heart-healing book, *Enchanted Love: The Mystical Power of Intimate Relationships*, bestselling author Marianne Williamson suggests, "Our wounds have been brought forward, not to block the experience of love, but to serve it."

We have all heard stories about people saying they won't ever be involved in a love relationship again. The wall goes up and the retreat begins. If you are retreating, why not advance instead? Why not work toward trusting that you are able to have healthy, intimate relationships? Why not practice by treating yourself how you want others to treat you? Make the choice to change the script from what it was in the past. What do you have to lose? What do you have to gain?

Intimacy can play a part in many kinds of relationships, not just romantic ones. The intimacy you have with your relationship to God gets deeper with prayer and meditation. It can remind you that you are never, ever alone. The treasures of intimacy found in the deep connection with a spouse, partner, dear friend, or relative can be profound.

When talking about intimacy, it brings up the importance of touch. Hugging can be a great way to connect through touch. Some people choose to hug with their heart touching the other person's heart. Some people are light huggers while others hold you like a bear. The warmth and connection of hugs are priceless. Use your wise judgment as to when it's appropriate to hug. Some people are uncomfortable or even startled by hugs, so when in doubt, ask, "May I give you a hug?" Honoring the answer is important and there's no need to take it personally if the person says no.

Embracing intimacy is a gift you give yourself. Your heart is much stronger than you may think. Do you want to create a bigger space in your heart for grace and love to enter? Allow intimacy to be a vibrant connection to your wisdom.

Tips for Welcoming More Intimacy Into Your Life

1. Love yourself a little bit more than you did yesterday. No big leaps; just increase your self-love by a smidgen, like dialing up to the next highest frequency on a radio. Many of us were taught that it was vain to love ourselves. If this is true for you, this may be a bit more challenging.

2. When you are ready, let go of the power and lingering pain stemming from any harsh words or treatment from family or friends that may have kept you in your own "unlovable"

category. (Note: do this only if you really want to . . .actually, some people find it's just easier to keep thinking they are unlovable. You have a choice.)

3. Name one thing you love or like about yourself. Start there. Remember, God doesn't make junk.

4. Dare to practice honest communication. Tell the truth with kindness, respect, and compassion.

5. Practice forgiveness. Forgive yourself and others—when you are ready. People who struggle with intimacy often carry heavy baggage filled with situations that are hard to forgive. When you're ready, and only when you are ready, put down the bags. Notice how you feel.

6. Give yourself the gift of professional support if you believe your intimacy issues keep you stuck in past beliefs. Anger, hurt, and past resentments stick to our "baggage" and are sometimes really, really hard to un-pack. You don't have to do this alone.

7. Pray, meditate, or seek spiritual support from God or whatever you call the Divine.

21

Love Radically

○ ○

And now these three remain: faith, hope and love. But the greatest of these is love.

—1 Corinthians 13:13

Years ago I gave my father a spice tin labeled "Love." At the time, he was lovingly taking over all of the cooking responsibilities as he nourished my mother in her final year of life. Printed at the bottom of the tin was the net weight "immeasurable"—and the list of ingredients included: joy, kindness, patience, peace, trust, and goodness, among other loving qualities. The directions for use encouraged the cook to add a big pinch of Love to every recipe. I believe my dad was adding a big dose of "radical love" to my mom's life in many sweet and tender ways. After my father passed away, I inherited this spice tin and use it frequently. It has a place of honor on my kitchen stove.

As you know, you don't need a spice tin to add love to food or to life. When I put my attention toward love, I find that it fills and deeply nourishes my mind, body, and spirit. This attention doesn't come from a place of seeking or longing, but rather it seems to be radically splashing out from me. As I splash, I have learned that love flows best when it flows freely, with no expectations attached. And in challenging situations when that flow feels blocked, I often ask, "What would love do now?"

The word *radical* means, "relating to or affecting the fundamental nature in something." Its synonyms are: fundamental, essential, deep-seated, sweeping, thorough, far-reaching, and major. What great sentiments to think about when deepening your thoughts on love, or commitment, or marriage.

A few years ago I was having a great conversation with a man I had just met. He mentioned that he was still friends with his former wife, despite the fact that their marriage had failed. After commenting on how awesome it was to still be friends with his former wife, I found myself telling him, "I've had two successful marriages!" I went on to say, "I've been divorced twice but I refuse to think of them as 'failed' marriages." I surprised myself, as it had taken me years to forgive myself for choosing to end the 25-year marriage to my high school sweetheart and a two-year marriage that followed some years later. Initially, I felt like I had a scarlet "D" on my forehead. I, Susan Tate, was Divorced. I was embarrassed and a bit ashamed that I couldn't make a marriage work "till death do us part." But as I healed my heart, I realized those two marriages were filled with love—radical love. I'm glad I was married.

And I wouldn't trade a day. These experiences were successful in taking me to the next level of learning and loving. I learned so much and I treasure and respect both marriages. I personally believe I had a sacred soul agreement with each of these amazing men. Do I wish I could have stayed married and reveling in the happily-ever-after? Of course, but that's not what life dealt and I don't regret my decisions. Did everyone work as hard as they could to save the marriages? My response is an unequivocal, "Yes." Now *that's* fundamental, essential, deep-seated, sweeping, thorough, far-reaching, and major love!

Speaking of radical love, I must admit that prior to my first divorce, I would judge people who couldn't stay married, couldn't make their marriage "successful"—and I too thought people and marriages had failed. I am still learning lessons of humility and non-judging. I was standing next to a good friend in her kitchen when she spoke about a woman we both knew: "She's on her third husband!" (A somewhat judgmental statement, just like I used to make.) She said it like that was some horrid damnable thing! "Bite your tongue!" I laughingly said to her. "I plan to be on my third husband some day!"

While we're on the topic of love, marriage, and commitment, I ecstatically recommend Elizabeth Gilbert's *Committed: A Skeptic Makes Peace with Marriage.*" She presents a history of marriage that is enlightening, captivating, and sometimes startling. Her personal navigation through her own belief system may prompt an expanded awareness of your own beliefs.

Marriage is sacred to me and I honor and value it. And sometimes marriages end, and it's healthier that way for everyone. And it hurts like hell (and by the way, no, I don't think I'm going there!) So, if your marriage or commitment to a life partner has ended, consider (in time) calling it a success. Love yourself. Love the other. Now, that's radical love, don't you think?

In other circumstances, it's quite easy to love. The words, "I love you" flow easily in my daily prayers as I send loving thoughts to my children, grandchildren, family, and friends. That's easy love. But for me, loving radically sometimes means loving people when they might not appear very loveable. It means sending love to terrorists and people I don't really like. It means sending love to the person at the post office who was wearing a hat to cover her hair loss from radiation treatments. It means loving myself as I am now, as I was before, and as the person I am becoming.

Radical love can also mean choosing love over fear. Do you have a steady hum of fear running through your mind? How would it feel to shift your fearful thinking to "love-full" thinking?

Cellular biologist Bruce Lipton, Ph.D., writes an attention-grabbing statement in his powerful work, *The Biology of Belief: Unleashing the Power of Consciousness, Matter and Miracles.* He states, "The simple truth is, when you're frightened you're dumber." Now I am not one to label someone's intelligence, but after reading his biological explanation of how our cells respond so unfavorably to a steady diet of fear, I believe I personally make healthier, smarter choices when choosing love rather than fear.

Dr. Lipton's statement doesn't refer to the instant rush of adrenaline or cortisol that floods our bloodstream when the "fight or flight" response kicks into gear as our body or mind perceives a fear-filled threat. This response is actually a built-in source of genetic wisdom that supports our quick reactions and decision-making that will hopefully keep us safe. In these instances, fear is a good thing, and the chemical reactions in the body are designed to support us in making smarter decisions.

Instead, Lipton's statement refers to a steady diet of fight/flight, over-activated by a build-up of excessive stress. That constant drain actually challenges our decision-making process and can lead to choices that probably aren't as smart as decisions we'd choose through the lens of love.

Overall, when we make decisions based on love rather than fear, our choices will be healthier, as well as smarter. When I view this concept through a political lens, it makes me respect our leaders who draw from the energy of love rather than fear. When I tune in to my business decisions, I want to be sure I am making grounded, intelligent, and loving choices for the good of all involved. In relationships, I want to speak from the chambers of my heart where I know love (radical love) and truth reside. In financial decision-making, I want to choose with intelligence and without the six-o'clock news scaring me with a constant forecast of economic or global gloom and doom.

Rev. Michael Bernard Beckwith expresses a powerful view of love in his words: "Love. You are not meant to search for it. You are not meant to wait for it. You are meant to generate it." Hmm, that could be my new definition of radical love.

Elisabeth Kübler-Ross said, "Make your decisions based on love, not fear." It is our choice. I want to love radically. Do you?

Here are seven action steps aimed at directing your thinking more toward radical love. Feel free to add more.

Seven Steps for Choosing (Radical) Love Over Fear

1. Lovingly observe when you enter the emotional realm of fearful thinking. You might say to yourself, "Ah, this is an opportunity for me to choose either fear or love. I choose love."

2. Take three deep, calming breaths when you notice stressful, physical sensations in your gut, the pit in your stomach,

your rapidly beating heart, or the tightness in your neck or back.

3. Practice mindfulness meditation.

4. Move your body. Walk, run, swim, dance, bike, do Nia, yoga, or Pilates. Physical exercise produces endorphins (providing a morphine-like high) right from your body's own personal pharmacy.

5. Pray, meditate, chant, or sing. Marianne Williamson wisely suggests that we place our fears and concerns "on the altar to be altered." I love that concept!

6. Extend love often and be the place where love shows up.

7. Generate and choose radical love every chance you get.

22

Enjoy Conscious Sexuality

○ ○

We can heal and strengthen ourselves during our conscious sexual activity, but we must know what we are doing and why.

—Iyanla Vanzant

Mindful, meaningful sexual activity can result in exquisite pleasure. This chapter is directed to those who choose to place their sexual beliefs in a high and holy place. Walt Whitman said, "If anything is sacred, the human body is sacred." I agree. We will explore this topic within the context of sacred, meaningful relationships—your relationship with yourself, as well as relationships with a partner.

Conscious is defined as being "awake and aware of one's surroundings and identity." To be conscious is to be intentional. To be awake and aware as we make sexual decisions can be quite a gift.

Sexuality is far more than just sex. I define *sex* as the physical acts of intimacy as it relates to your sexuality. *Sexuality* is a broader term that includes an intricate combination of biological, ethical, cultural, and psychological dimensions. It includes your values, spiritual and religious beliefs, gender identity, sexual orientation, customs, self-concept, attitudes, behaviors, and much, much more.

To enjoy conscious sex and sexuality, we need to know how to make choices that honor us as well as our partners. We need to be in the present moment yet aware of the gifts or consequences of our actions.

We need to honor our spiritual beliefs. We need to be honest. We need to *know* what we are saying *yes* to.

Conscious sexuality begins with our intimate relationship with our own bodies. Our thoughts and perceptions about sexuality directly affect our experiences. Do you feel guilt or shame when you touch, or even look at, your own genitals? The word "masturbation" is a term that is traditionally loaded with negativity. You might choose to use the term "self-pleasuring" instead, as it bypasses guilt, shame, and blame. I think this trio of beliefs has done a great deal of harm to our thoughts about sexuality. Medical professionals suggest that it is perfectly normal to privately touch your body in a pleasing way. It's also normal to not touch yourself.

When I was a young mother, one of my friends took her three-year-old son, Nicholas, to the doctor for his well-child exam. She told the doctor that her little boy was often touching his penis and she wondered if this was okay. The doctor grinned as he replied, "Linda, it feels good! Let him do it!"

Self-pleasuring is an intimate, private behavior. Once we know how to pleasure ourselves, it's easier to help our partner know how to please us too. Pleasuring our bodies can be a gift of appreciation—and as the doctor said, "It feels good!"

Sharing sexual intimacy with a partner has the potential to take both people to a place of deep soul communion. Consciously communicating your likes and dislikes to your beloved is a skill that may not come naturally. Having the intention to practice this kind of intimate communication will deeply nourish your mind, body and spirit. Telling your partner "I really like it when you touch me here" is an easy guiding phrase. Or, you might say, "I feel uncomfortable when you do that" to communicate what you don't want. Avoiding sentences with the "accusatory you" will go far to strengthen intimate communication. If you find yourself beginning a sentence with accusations like, "You always ..." or "You never ...", the other person probably won't feel like staying around to hear the rest of your sentence. Talking to each other about sex (another form of oral sex!) and listening to each other with love, appreciation, and openness, can provide a connection that adds delight, joy, closeness, and tenderness to your relationship. Participating in honest, loving, and intimate communication then, is quintessential foreplay.

Not everyone feels comfortable discussing sex or sexuality. In the nineties I was the consultant for a cooperative grant with the CDC and the American College Health Association. I was able to travel across the United States to provide training for college professors on how to teach education majors how to teach about HIV and AIDS in their classrooms. I remember one of my colleagues sharing a story about her grandmother asking her about the AIDS education work she had been doing. Her grandmother said, "All this talk about oral sex! I just don't understand how *talking* about AIDS can transmit it!" My colleague consciously chose not to provide details.

Think back to how you learned about sexuality. Was it an open, sacred, pleasurable, confident experience? When I ask this type of question at workshops or other presentations, approximately 10 percent of the people raise their hands. Most of those are under the age of 30, so things are improving. When I first asked the question in the seventies, rarely did anyone raise a hand.

There was a time when I felt some anger toward my mother for not being more open with me on this topic. It took me until age 40 to realize that she couldn't have been any different in sharing information about this topic. No one really had been open with her. And in some way, it's why I am so passionate about sharing the concept of sacred and pleasurable sexuality. Wow, sacred and pleasurable in the same sentence!

Parents have a wonderful opportunity to provide high and holy sexuality education from infancy. Valuing females as equally as males is a good start. Teaching children the proper names for penis and vagina would be another early part of the process. Adults still giggle as they come up with silly words for genitals. We don't make up goofy words for elbow or nose, so why do we change the names for parts "down there"? Maybe it is because no one taught us with clarity and a calm truth.

Back for a moment to the concept of self-pleasuring. Most children find out how much fun it is to touch their penis or rub their clitoris at an early age. An overwhelming majority of adults have told me that they had their hand smacked or were yelled at the first time they were "caught" in this pleasurable act. I've heard of other parents who've been able to provide a positive response that has supported a healthy and beautiful attitude about sex that lasts throughout life. I know of one 7-year-old child who sweetly said to her mother, "Oh, Mom, when I touch myself here it feels so good that sometimes I feel like I'm going to explode!" This mother answered her daughter in a way that I would imagine would help this little girl grow into adulthood with a strong sense of enjoying conscious sexuality. The mother, in my opinion, had a brilliant and loving reply: "Isn't it wonderful?" she said. "That part of your body is so special!" She went on to tell her daughter that touching her clitoris is something that's private, and something she would want to do in her bedroom when no one is around.

The Dagara tribe in West Africa does not have words for "having sex." Their language equivalent is "going on a journey together." Conscious sexuality can be a wondrous journey. Choosing to honor our bodies and to act in a mindful manner can add much joy and satisfaction to this sacred part of our lives. Kahlil Gibran wrote, "And your body is the harp of your soul, And it is yours to bring forth sweet music from it or confused sounds." Enjoy your melody!

Seven Sacred Ways to Ecstatically Enjoy Conscious Sexuality

1. Know what you are saying yes to.

2. Treat your body like the temple it is.

3. Love, explore, and know your body. Keep it as healthy as possible. Know what kind of touch turns you on. Practice and enjoy touching yourself if that feels right to you. If you have a partner, ask what turns him or her on. If it's comfortable for both of you, doesn't hurt anyone, and honors your spiritual beliefs, try it!

4. When and if you are ready, forgive anyone who caused you sexual pain and suffering. Incest, rape, and abuse are horrid crimes that leave unseen marks on the soul. There are amazing stories of people who have survived and even

thrived after traveling their own healing path to the other side of the pain. Seek professional and divine support. You deserve to ecstatically enjoy conscious sexuality.

5. If you have a beloved partner, revel in honest and intimate communication. Enjoy being thankful for the results. Tenderly and truthfully expressing what you sexually like or don't like can be the best foreplay and after-play there is.

6. Orgasms don't last as long as foreplay and the after-glow. Revel in it all!

7. Enjoy deepening your connection to your body as a sacred vessel of love and pleasure. Remain awake and aware as you consciously make, and then evaluate, your sexual decisions.

23

Honor Orgasms

○ ○

The extent to which we deny our spirituality we limit our sexuality; the extent to which we judge our sexuality we limit our spirituality. Here, orgasm is the teacher.
—Kenneth Ray Stubbs

Orgasms are marvelous gifts—as blessed to give as to receive. As a sexuality educator for almost four decades, I've heard many people (all female) share their concern that they weren't having orgasms or were not sure what they felt like. I believe this concern is often fueled by the magazines that create this angst through articles entitled, "How good a lover are you?" or "Test your orgasm IQ." This sometimes sets people up for a sense of failure. Everyone wants to compare. We all have asked the question, "Am I normal?"

Orgasms, for men, are usually obvious. The ejaculation of semen signals the finale of a group of muscular contractions that have heightened to a point of release. Orgasms for women are different in that they may not always be quite so apparent. They vary in intensity and may feel subtle at times or more vigorous at other times. Sometimes that leaves a woman wondering if she's even had an orgasm.

I strongly believe that the most important sexual organ is not between the legs; it's between the ears. In sexuality, as in other parts of our lives, our thoughts help to create our reality. Sex can be as good as you think it can be. If your partner is lying there agonizing or analyzing whether or not he or she did "it" right (according to some random magazine sexual IQ test) it can take you out of the present moment. What's right is right for you if it doesn't hurt anyone and is in line with your spiritual and/or religious beliefs.

Speaking of orgasms and religious beliefs in the same sentence . . . if you ever doubt the divine plan in all this, just think about how many people often cry out "Oh God! Oh God!" during the exquisite delight orgasmic bliss . . .

When I was a professor at the University of Virginia, I was interviewed for a *60 Minutes* segment along with students from my *Sexuality Today* class. Mike Wallace's producer asked the students if I had ever specifically taught them the mechanics of having sex. Kelly, a 21-year-old student, answered the question beautifully, saying that I had taught them everything that could or should happen before sex (including communication, decision-making, and choosing protection) and everything that could or should happen after sexual intimacy. She said I taught them that if the couple concentrated on doing those things in a way that was honoring and respecting each other, that whatever happened during the actual act of sex was just right for that couple; therefore I didn't need to teach them the "mechanical" aspects of sex. I wanted to jump on top of the table and cheer! She clearly understood the heart of how I teach about sexuality.

Honor your own orgasms if you choose to self-pleasure. Know that some people touch themselves and others don't. Both choices are normal. (I did need to remind the high school students I taught years ago that it was *not* appropriate to be touching yourself as you walked down the hall ...) If you have a partner, revel in the other person's orgasms and don't feel you need to have them simultaneously or a certain way. Every person is unique; every expression of sexuality is different than the one before.

Knowing what makes you feel good can be communicated to your partner. If you are not comfortable giving verbal directions, gently move your partner's hands, fingers, or mouth where you want them to be (and be sure that's comfortable for them to do). Orgasms and sexuality can be fun, sacred, splendid, messy, silly, and so awesome!

Remember to nurture your most important sexual organ (the brain), cultivate positive thoughts, and weed out the destructive or painful ones. You have a choice of how you think. You have a choice to really enjoy the gift of orgasm and the gifts of glorious sexuality. The dictionary defines honor as "having high respect for or glory." Do you treat your body with glory and high respect? Honoring your sexuality and your orgasms deserves a place of high respect. Honor on!

Five Enticing Ways to Honor Orgasms

1. Practice.

2. Enjoy.

3. Practice some more.

4. Seek pleasure.

5. Okay, Okay, I know you're looking for more "how-tos" here. So, I would suggest you get a copy of *The Illustrated Guide to Extended Massive Orgasm* by Steve and Vera Bodansky. The Amazon.com description summarizes the book well: "Written for men and women, straight and gay, the book graphically, playfully, and sensually discusses the best hand and body positions, the enticements of teasing and begging, and the subtle intricacies of peaking and coming down." Enjoy! And I do mean, enjoy!

24

Be a Good Receiver

○ ○
It is by giving that we receive.

—*Luke 6:38*

I am discovering that people often fall into one of these two categories—they are either a very good giver or a very good receiver. In an unscientific study, I've noticed that most people are usually better givers than receivers. It makes us feel good to do things for other people. Yet often when we are "given back to" in the form of a "thank you" we attempt to deflect it. If someone picks up the check to buy your lunch, do you protest? If someone compliments you on a job well done, do you shrug it off? I'm learning that accepting gifts, compliments, and support with a gracious and meaningful "thank you" completes the circle of giving. It also honors and respects the person who has offered this gift.

In other words, it's as important to receive as it is to give. Now, some people may get carried away with this concept and just sit back with their hands out to receive (take?) all the time. That's not what I'm talking about here. Sometimes we may feel the need to be the constant giver, too. I think that need often indicates a discomfort in receiving or possibly a wish that we might be liked more for always giving. Do you feel deserving to receive your good? You are. You are deserving of all good.

You may want to notice, throughout the next few days, how you give and how you receive. Do you give freely without expectations? Do you receive graciously, accepting your good and the other person's gift to you? Do you give more than you receive? Do you receive more than you give?

Giving and receiving with ease can add to your sense of well-being and be truly nourishing. Enjoy being a generous giver. Enjoy being a gracious receiver.

Tips for Expanding Your Ability to Receive

1. Explore your mental conditioning as it relates to receiving. Were you taught it was a bit selfish or egotistical to accept praise? Well, it's not. Examine the possibility that giving and receiving are equally honorable.

2. The next time you receive a compliment, simply say, "Thank you!" and let the words sink in as you fully receive, rather than deflect, the gift you have been given. This is such a beautiful way to acknowledge the person and the gift.

3. Observe (without judging) how others accept praise or thanks.

4. Consider the possibility that giving and receiving are as inextricably linked as inhaling and exhaling.

25

Eliminate Clutter

○ ○
Our life is frittered away by detail . . . simplify, simplify.
—*Henry David Thoreau*

Anyone familiar with the metaphysical law that deals with clearing out space in order to receive more has experienced the joy of what happens after you eliminate clutter. I'm not talking about the minimal amount of "clutter" that will always be part of life, but the clutter that gets overwhelming, takes up too much space or time, and really doesn't add to the beauty and ease of your life. One of the most freeing things I have ever done was to abolish unnecessary clutter. And believe me, I know what clutter looks like. More good things can come into your life when you've created a place for them to enter.

If you are ready to face the challenge of getting rid of things you really don't need or use, I suggest you start small. Open your clothes closet. (Okay, this might not be small, but I didn't mention the attic or garage yet.) Allocate a set amount of time for this project and then separate the clothes you wear from the clothes you haven't worn in the past year or two. I did this many years ago when my inspiration was twofold: 1) I was moving from Virginia to the Pacific Northwest and 2) there was a local women's shelter collecting clothing. I found it easier to give up clothes that I really liked but just wasn't wearing anymore when I could donate to someone in need.

The next step is to take another closet, drawer, or bookshelf and go to it. When you're ready, delete old e-mail files and clean out your car. The physical and mental space that it clears is worth your time. Recycling and donating also makes you feel good.

I find the amount of clutter around the house has a distinct correlation to the amount of emotional clutter going on in the head. Is that true for you? Sometimes we fill up those spaces so we don't have to process that stuff and it just bonks around in our heads without any movement forward. Things just can't move anywhere in all that clutter!

Now that you've done a closet or a drawer or two, it's time to tackle the potentially overwhelming part—the memorabilia. What to keep and what to throw out can vary through the years, but it may be worth the time to sort through some of these things on occasion.

A real turning point for me in this area was when we sold my parents' home after my mother's death and had the task of packing up 53 years of a household. My sentimental mother saved every card my dad had ever sent to her, every card she sent to him, every card she received from her 5 children, 15 grandchildren, 13 great grandchildren . . . well, you get the idea. It was like a Hallmark card factory. My siblings and I couldn't possibly go through all of the memorabilia so we carefully selected a few favorites and we recycled the rest. Well, actually, if memory serves, my sister Beth temporarily recycled the rest to her house.

Speaking of Beth, I must add that we did need to restrain her from unhinging the kitchen door she wanted to include in her pile of memories. The heights of all the Tate children and their children were marked on that door and she was determined to take it with her! She also agonized a bit over who should get the Dalmatian dog toilet brush holder.

The first night I arrived home to begin this overwhelming task, I sat by myself in the living room and gazed at all that was around me. There was the family Bible on the table by my dad's favorite chair, my mom's music box collection, a small bust of Jackie Kennedy, family photographs on the dining room wall, and the old maple stereo console we'd had since the sixties. Anticipating the next four days of packing and removing remnants of our family's life together in this house, I began to cry. It seemed like a task I was too young to be doing and nothing seemed to make any sense. How would it feel to never come home again?

After praying for a few minutes, I felt a deep sense of peace wash over me. Spirit was clearly at work here, as I felt I was receiving a profound gift that enabled me to move through this passage with grace, strength, and trust. This gift proved to be more valuable than any household item in our lovely family home. I realized that it wasn't the stuff, it wasn't the dishes, and it wasn't the doors or the walls or my old bedroom that was important at that moment. It wasn't the living room where I stood for photos in my prom and wedding dresses or groaned when mom wanted to take one more family picture. It wasn't the things—it was the space in between that was important. The gift was the realization that the *space in between* all this stuff was where I had learned to love. And that love was something I was able to safely pack with me and keep for the rest of my life. My tears stopped and I thanked God for the gift of this peaceful insight, and for the gift of such loving parents.

After that extended weekend of overwhelming memories, I went home and pulled out my stash of Hallmark treasures—the wedding cards, birthday cards (the apple doesn't fall very far from the tree), and early artwork from the children. I created a memory box for both of our children and filled it with special treasures. I then fashioned my own box and mindfully sorted through what things had the most meaning for me. It felt so cleansing. I was able to keep memories but not as much memorabilia. I didn't need 20 cards from my fortieth birthday or the get-well cards from years ago to remind me of my past surgeries and illnesses. Someone once told me that if you have something special that you love so much, either hang it in the living room so you can see it every day or get rid of it! What an interesting concept.

Traveling lighter feels luscious. I continue to create new memories and treasure each event but I more consciously choose what gets recycled back into the universe. As you eliminate clutter and simplify, you will know what to keep and what to share.

Twelve Tips to Reduce Clutter
(Note: Pick 2 then come back and pick 2 more when you're ready!)

1. Start small. Create 15 minutes to clean and organize just one drawer.

2. Decide what charity or consignment store you would like to receive the clothes and household items you no longer use.

3. Sort mail each day. Have a place for your bills (including online files as well as tangible paper files). Have a box for junk mail so it can be shredded later.

4. Take 10 minutes to delete old e-mails. Then, take another 10 minutes when it feels right!

5. Put this book down and put away 5 things in their correct place. Don't forget to come back to read the next tip!

6. Consider giving away or recycling one thing for every piece of clothing or household item you bring into your home.

7. If you're unsure whether you are ready to release something, put it in a box and store it in the garage, attic, or closet. A year later when you realize you haven't used it, pass it on.

8. If you have school-aged children, create a box for each of them so you can save special papers, photos, and projects.

9. Group things together that go together: office supplies, cleaning products, winter gloves, etc.

10. Decide what part of your clutter bothers you the most, put on some fun music, and go to it.

11. Ask others in your household to come up with organizational tips that would benefit everyone.

12. Don't fret. Give up the idea that one day everything will be in its proper place. Really, how boring would that be? Create

open, clean, energetic places whenever you can and do the best you can. We never get it all done. Ah, what a relief!

26

Be a Lifelong Learner

Nothing can dim the light that shines from within.
—Maya Angelou

The intellectual path of wellness is expansive. A trip to the library for a book or downloading the latest bestseller on a Kindle can add a little spark of excitement to the part of your brain that constantly seeks to learn new things. It seems the older we get the more time we have to learn. Many elders take advantage of lifelong learning by taking free courses or finding creative ways to travel. I imagine they are probably more intellectually stimulated than those who have stopped to pause along the way. So many young people today are traveling abroad, learning specific trades and skills, taking college classes, investing time and attention to the arts—and are delving deeply into the pleasures of learning.

During her sophomore year at Beloit College, my daughter Molly was able to schedule a semester abroad in Senegal. I knew Senegal was in West Africa but didn't know much else about the land, the people, or the culture there. I went to the library and brought home several books that helped me to learn more. One of them was a children's book that was a quick read; pages full of photos were much more exciting than pages full of small print. I read the children's book cover to cover and scanned the others. It felt so good to be able to talk to Molly and sound somewhat intelligent about the place where she would be living for several months. During one of our phone conversations, she astutely asked me if I had just come from the library. She had a pretty strong intuition that I hadn't always known that Wolof was the language spoken there or that Dakar was the capital!

You can enjoy the library or press a button on your computer to access more information than you could ever absorb in your lifetime. The choices expand when you add classes or travel or crossword puzzles or anything that keeps your brain cells dancing!

So, keep your brain actively stimulated by always reaching out to learn something new. There is a bright light shining within each of us and we can keep it beaming through our lifelong learning process. This is an invigorating way to add to our wellness wisdom. What are you doing this week that helps to expand your learning?

Enjoyable Ways to Expand Your Lifelong Learning Opportunities

1. Read. Always have fresh books or even previously read books available to read or to listen to—and enjoy.

2. Take a class to learn something absolutely new. Choose something that feels exciting so you'll enjoy the learning process.

3. Journal your thoughts and add your wisdom to the mix.

4. Enroll in a continuing education class. You may want to consider asking a good friend to join you.

5. Create or join a book discussion group.

27

Take a Well Day

○ ○

Imagine taking a day to be guided solely by pure delight.
—Charlotte Davis Kasl

What would our work lives be like if we had the opportunity to take "well days" off from work instead of sick days? I believe we would have less illness and more energy to use more productively at our jobs and at home. Of course, we would need some provision for the unexpected illness or injury too. But it seems if we took a day here and there to celebrate our wellness, to practice self-care, to take a one day mini-vacation, to stay in bed, to read, to write, to walk, to be alone, or to be with a special someone—that our overall level of wellness would benefit greatly.

Why not suggest a new employment benefit to be negotiated the next time the opportunity arises? Many enlightened employers already offer this benefit. If you have a certain number of sick days allotted, encourage a few of them to be designated as well days. Changing the consciousness in businesses, schools, and corporations doesn't happen overnight, but gentle changes can occur if more people gather with the intent of improving life for everyone. It takes being bold and standing up for yourself. Tap into your wellness wisdom for strategies that can result in positive changes for many. If you are self-employed or are a full-time parent or caregiver, it may be even more important to create well days in your schedule. You deserve it. Why not plan on giving yourself a well day soon?

Things To Do on Your Well Day

1. Sleep in as late as you can or take a nap mid-day if that appeals to you.

2. Schedule something to do that will absolutely provide pleasure.

3. Prepare or buy a special food that nourishes and delights you.

4. Create time to enjoy a physical activity your body loves.

5. Set aside 15 minutes to get something done that would be great to cross off your to do list.

28

Practice Mindfulness

○ ○
Wherever you go, there you are.

—Jon Kabat-Zinn

Jon Kabat-Zinn, founder and director of the Stress Reduction Clinic at the University of Massachusetts Medical Center, defines *mindfulness* as "paying attention in a particular way; on purpose, in the present moment, and non-judgmentally. This kind of attention nurtures greater awareness, clarity, and acceptance of present-moment reality."

Mindfulness is a state of present-moment-ness that brings everything we're doing into a place of focus. We can make love, eat, talk, walk, work, drive, sing, or pray mindfully. Isn't it interesting that we might need to practice such a concept?

Would you like to practice right now? You can do this with any food, but I'm going to describe the experience of eating a raisin with mindfulness.

Mindful Eating Meditation

Take a raisin in your hand. Now touch it and gently roll it in between your fingertips. Feel its texture. See its texture and the color and the shape and the patterns of the wrinkles in that raisin. Now put it up to your nose and smell it. Absorb the aroma. Think back to every event that had to take place so that this raisin is now able to be in your hand. The soil in the vineyards was prepared and the grape vines were delicately planted. The sun and rain provided nourishment for growth. In time, workers picked the grapes, dried them, packed them and then shipped them off to your neighborhood store. You then purchased the raisins and brought them home. Now, you have one in your hand.

Gently place the raisin on your tongue. Without chewing, just feel it there. Move it around all over your mouth. Slowly, consciously begin to chew. Feel the first squish; notice the taste and sensations you experience. Chew it as long as you can, enjoying each movement of your mouth and tongue. Finally, swallow the raisin, noticing how wonderful it is to have the ability to swallow—a very natural function of the human body.

There, you have eaten a raisin with mindfulness. How did that feel? Was the experience richer because of your mindfulness? Can you sip a glass of juice or eat an orange the same way? Can you eat a salad or a delicious dessert with the same awareness? Try eating one meal in a slower, more mindful way. You may develop a new appreciation for the food or even discover that you don't like what you're eating. Your body's ability to chew, swallow, and digest need not be taken for granted.

Mindfulness can be practiced in all areas of your life. You will be graced with the gentle pleasure of present moment peace that comes with turning your attention to what it is you are doing right now.

A mindful walk (or roll if you move with a Segway or wheelchair) might be the next thing to incorporate. Practicing mindfulness in different parts of our life can deepen and broaden experiences. Mindfulness usually leads to less stress and a more peaceful way of thinking and feeling. Enjoy the practice—mindfully—as you transform this concept into your expanding wellness wisdom.

29

Live in the Present Moment

○ ○ ○ ○ ○ ○ ○ ○ ○ ○ ○ ○ ○ ○ ○ ○ ○ ○ ○ ○

Breathing in, I calm my body.
Breathing out, I smile.
Dwelling in the present moment,
I know this is a wonderful moment!
—Thich Nhat Hanh

Living in the present moment is a glorious—yet sometimes challenging—concept. Many of us spend endless hours worrying about the future or fretting about the past. Why not stop for a moment and notice all the great things going on in your life this second? Notice your breath, your heartbeat and your senses. It's an easy way to settle into this very moment. Notice the fact that you have made the decision to take time to read a book all about enhancing wellness for *you*. Reveling in the what's-good-about-this-moment can cause much bliss.

In his acclaimed bestseller, *The Power of Now*, Eckhart Tolle suggests that we can find more joy in our lives if we keep our thinking out of the past or future and focus on the *now*. ET (my new affectionate name for Eckhart Tolle, since ET has clearly called my soul home!) suggests that we cause ourselves more pain by resisting the present moment. Byron Katie, another author-sage, states simply, "What is, is." If we can accept all that is contained in "what is" in the present moment, our lives could be quite peaceful. This kind of awareness would let us know that the painful moments will pass.

Being conscious of our breath is one way to access the present moment. Breath can immediately take you to a more centered place and offer a way of connecting you to your inner wisdom. Deep, easy belly breathing can result in a feeling of relaxation that provides a steady fuel for daily activities.

If we pause to mindfully focus on our breath, we can help release anxious or fearful feelings, calm our thoughts, and better access the present moment. The breath is always available for us to use as a tool to "get back home" to our inner selves. The present really is a gift you give yourself.

Would you like to enjoy a minute or two of gentle belly breathing? It may gift you with more awareness of the present moment.

Gentle Belly Breathing Meditation

Just notice the air as it travels in through your nose, expands your belly and lungs, and then leaves your body and is released again through the nostrils. Place your hands on your belly and watch and feel it rise and fall as you breathe in and out. Gently add more breath as you inhale to extend the belly and the chest and then pause before you fully exhale. Take ten beautiful breaths. In your mind you can simply say "in" on the in breath and "out" on the out breath. Feel free to smile as you practice this calming technique that softly expands your awareness of the present moment.

30

Don't Complain

I can't complain, but sometimes I still do.

—Joe Walsh

How would your life be different if you stopped complaining? Do you dare to try it? What would you need to give up if you did? I had to give up receiving people's sympathy for "poor me." After years of a series of dramatic life events, it was challenging to give up this attention. I actually got pretty good at acting strong while still giving off the oh-woe-is-me vibe! But the gift of positive energy that flows and actually blasts all around you when you stop the complaining is quite worth it. I no longer feel like a victim of any of my life's circumstances. I am increasingly attentive to my words and thoughts, and strive to speak in a manner that constantly creates a vision of what I want my life to be.

I am not suggesting that you be stoic and hide your feelings. I am suggesting that you take a look at the problem but turn your attention toward a solution or reframe the situation. Let's take something simple like the weather. I know people that celebrate the snow, bless the rain, and just go about enjoying whatever the day brings. I know others who moan about the rain, the cold, the heat, or the wind. I live in Seattle where some folks (just a few) dwell on the often gray and overcast skies. On that type of day, most Seattleites I know see the time of day when the sun appears. We actually call them "sun breaks" here! They notice the sunny parts of the day—not the dreary ones. Do you tend to see the clouds or the sun?

Observe, just for a day, your own complaint talk. Does it affect your sense of wellness? Does it make it more enjoyable? Now, try going through a week without complaining. It brings life's challenges, big and small, to an easier level when you can reframe those whiny words. If you're really ready for more wonderful experiences to enter your life, refrain from complaining for 21 days in a row! The universe gives us pretty much what we talk about and "order," so why not order up what you want with those words, rather than complaining about what you don't want or don't have?

Another self-check involves our talk of illness and injury. Do you begin many sentences with a description of you as your illness? "Oh, my allergies are flaring up again." "My bursitis is killing me." "My migraines are acting up." You are not your allergies, your cancer, your diabetes, your fibromyalgia, or your bipolar disorder. You are not your illness! If you have a minor, chronic or major illness, try going through the morning without mentioning it. Then try a whole day. Notice the difference in your discomfort or pain level. Why not trade those complaining words for healing ones?

It is okay and even necessary to express your needs or concerns. If you are feeling sick and need help, ask for what you need. If the hotel shower water comes out cold, it's perfectly right to call down to the front desk to request hot water. If someone is chewing on ice and the noise is irritating, kindly ask him if he can find a quieter way to enjoy his ice. Make your requests known without loading them with whining.

Visionary peace leader Marshall Rosenberg presents a powerful method of communicating needs in his well known work, *Nonviolent Communication: A Language of Life*. Dr. Rosenberg provides insights on how important it is to acknowledge our needs. He presents a model for language that results in a style of life-serving communication that is clear, honoring, and loving. Incorporating his concepts can result in an endless wellspring of enhanced, non-complaining communication that creates more harmony in your relationships.

Are you planning a trip? Announce the expectation to your traveling companions that the complaint department is closed during this holiday. Another suggestion is to request the dinner hour as a non-complaining time. This simple act of not complaining will add to your feelings of peace, joy, and contentment. It also can provide a healthy dose of nourishment for your mind, body, and spirit.

Are you ready to give up complaining? The rewards are great.

Five Suggestions to Support You in Implementing the Ideas in This Chapter

1. Observe, just for a day, your own complaint talk. Don't judge it; just be aware of it.

2. Notice if or when you include the word "my" in front of a health condition. Lovingly re-state and reframe your "my" thought. An example "My headache is killing me" might be reframed to "The tightness in my head is beginning to subside as I slow my breathing."

3. Ask for what you need in a clear, honoring, and loving manner. Don't assume those around you can read your mind.

4. Ask your family if they would support the idea of having meal times as a complaint-free time. This doesn't mean they can't express concerns of the day; it would just include an awareness of no whining or complaining as they share.

5. Don't complain. Notice how much better you feel.

31

Magnify Gratitude

○ ○
*Expressing gratitude ignites the light within us and is a
sure path to joy.*

—Charlotte Kasl

Adopting a conscious attitude of gratitude can bring increased joy into
our lives. Remember, what we focus on expands! Oft-quoted Meister
Eckhart, the medieval Christian mystic, said, "If the only prayer you
say in your life is 'thank you,' that would suffice."

Gratitude for what we have makes us appreciate everything even
more. If you awaken in the morning and give thanks for the sky, the
birds, the air, the wind, the rain, your heart beating, your ability to
breathe, the people in your life—the list is endless—you can't help but
to step into a more joyous day.

My former husband told me more than once, "It's hard to stay sad
when you're *in gratitude*." He was right. I've tried switching my thoughts
to gratitude when sadness gets overwhelming and it works for me. It
doesn't eliminate the sadness or its cause, but I've learned that if I take
time to observe and feel the sadness, I can then move away from the
painful thoughts through that doorway of gratitude. The more things
we are thankful for, the more things to be thankful for will show up
in our lives.

Taking time to craft a hand-written letter of gratitude to someone
for their kindness is an act that makes at least two people feel great.
Please don't wait for Thanksgiving to consider writing a gratitude letter

to a family member, co-worker, or friend. E-mail works too, but there's something special about receiving a hand-written letter, especially if it was penned with gratitude.

You may want to consider keeping a gratitude journal by your bed. Making a gratitude list at bedtime can help to create a peace-filled sleep, as well as become a wonderful addition to your spiritual practice. Or, you may just choose to close your eyes and rather than count sheep, count all of the things that happened that day that created gratitude.

Several years ago, my friend Roberta gave me a small circle of ten beautiful beads. Each night, I gently touch each bead and say "thank you" for a specific person or event that day. Her simple gift has provided a great way for me to magnify gratitude and it invariably sends me into a peaceful sleep.

The Rev. Dr. Michael Beckwith, founder of the Agape International Spiritual Center in California, shared a powerful statement about gratitude during his 2007 guest appearance on *Oprah*. He was discussing the Law of Attraction as he said, "Nothing new can come into your life until you are grateful for what you already have." You may want to read that sentence again.

Celebrating and magnifying gratitude is a wonderful practice that brightens the light of wellness wisdom that resides within each of us. With gratitude as your guide, I invite you to laugh, love, play, and pray your way into the continued nourishment of your mind, body, and spirit. Honor your wellness wisdom within.

Thank you for taking the time to read this book. I am grateful for you.

Ways to Magnify Gratitude

1. Start the day by giving thanks. As you open your eyes, you might say, "Thank you God! I get another day!"

2. Don't complain. The universe typically provides us with more of what we speak or think about each day. So the more you complain, the more you'll find reasons to complain! The more gratitude you acknowledge, more things to be grateful for will appear in your life.

3. Consider keeping a gratitude journal. Having a gratitude journal by your bed and writing just a few things in it each night can be a beautiful closure to the day.

4. If journaling isn't your thing, call to mind ten things you are grateful for before drifting off to sleep.

5. Write and send thank you notes, not just for something given to you recently but to acknowledge appreciation for something someone did for you in the past.

6. Don't wait for Thanksgiving or a special holiday to express gratitude, love, or appreciation to those you love. Call someone now. You'll make at least two people feel better.

7. Consider gratitude as a way of being. The suggestions above offer things *to do* that are supportive in developing the practice of gratitude. The next step is to know you can go even deeper and allow yourself *to be* the place where gratitude flourishes.

Closing Thoughts

So where do you want to go from here? You have the inspiration, theory, tools, affirmations, reflection pages, a Wellness Bill of Rights, and an action plan at your finger tips. One of the great things about wellness is its expansive and ever-changing nature. You can choose to add more at any time. You can add more love, forgiveness, gratitude, trust, movement, prayer, pleasure, laughter—the list goes well beyond the 31 concepts presented in this book.

You are invited to use these ideas as a guide; a blueprint for what wellness could look like for you. You are the architect. Create the body you love living in and nurture its foundation with the qualities that suit your way of living.

My desire is for you to use these ideas to nourish your mind, body, and spirit in the most joyful ways imaginable. In closing, I have written this prayer for you.

My Prayer for You

May you make wise choices that nourish your mind, body, and spirit.

May you see the infinite possibilities that exist with each sunrise.

May you allow your soul the freedom to express who you really are.

May you allow yourself to love greatly and be greatly loved.

May you know that good self-care ultimately supports all those around you.

May you discover peace-filled solutions in the opportunities of conflict.

May you allow yourself time to grieve.

May you use your gifts and talents to create a better world.

May you listen to others with ears of compassion.

May you forgive yourself and others for any behaviors or beliefs that have caused pain.

May you feel God's presence in every cell of your body.

May you be filled with gratitude for your daily blessings.

May you be well.

Amen.

Affirmations for Wellness

I accept balance in all aspects of me; including my mental, physical, spiritual, and emotional self.

I am enough.

Every cell in my body vibrates with health.

I forgive myself and I forgive others for any behaviors or beliefs that have caused pain.

I release and bless all thoughts and beliefs that no longer serve my highest purpose.

God is at home in me.

I am filled with gratitude for the abundant blessings I constantly receive from Spirit.

I allow myself to love greatly and be greatly loved.

I am constantly discovering my joy and it is powerful.

I am surrounded by feelings of harmony and peace.

I accept and receive all of my good now.

I lovingly accept joyful health to flow in and through my body.

I accept radiant health and wholeness.

I am a generous giver and a gracious receiver.

I commit to taking more time each day to be silent and still.

I know that *now* is the God moment.

I express my emotions with authenticity and clarity.

I speak with kindness, truth, and compassion.

I joyfully live a life full of integrity.

I mindfully choose my response to any circumstance or condition.

I am grateful for my body.

I revel in wholeness.

Wellness Action Plan

If we did all the things we are capable of doing, we would literally astonish ourselves.

~Thomas Edison

Before completing this action plan, first take a few breaths and then ask yourself these two questions: If you don't make any changes in your life, what will your life look like five years from now? Where do you want to be five years from now?

1. State your goal or intention and WHY you want it.

2. Are you ready to allow what you want to come into your life?

3. How will you know you will have reached your goal? List three things that will have occurred.

4. What small step can you take today to reach your goal?

5. What three steps will you take in the next few weeks to continue to work toward your goal?

Signature_____

Date_____

Bibliography

Beckwith, Michael Bernard. *Spiritual Liberation: Fulfilling Your Soul's Potential.* New York: Atria Books and Hillsboro, OR: Beyond Words, 2008.

Bodansky, Steve, and Vera Bodansky. *The Illustrated Guide to Extended Massive Orgasm.* Alameda, CA: Hunter House, 2002.

Borysenko, Joan. *A Woman's Journey to God.* New York: Riverhead Books, 1999.

—. *Minding the Body, Mending the Mind.* New York: Bantam Books, 1988.

Chopra, Deepak. *Quantum Healing: Exploring the Frontiers of Mind/Body Medicine.* New York: Bantam Books, 1989.

David, Marc. *The Slow Down Diet: Eating for Pleasure, Energy, & Weight Loss.* Rochester, VT: Healing Arts Press, 2005.

—. *Nourishing Wisdom: A Mind-Body Approach to Nutrition and Well-Being.* New York: Bell Tower, 1992.

"Discovering the Secret: How to Live the Secret." *The Oprah Winfrey Show.* NBC. 8 Feb. 2007. Television.

Dyer, Wayne W. *Manifest Your Destiny: The Nine Spiritual Principles for Getting Everything You Want.* New York: HarperCollins, 1997.

Friedman, Peach. *Diary of an Exercise Addict.* Guilford, CT: GPP Life, 2010.

Gilbert, Elizabeth. *Eat, Pray, Love.* New York: Penguin Books, 2006.

—. *Committed: A Skeptic Makes Peace with Marriage.* New York: Viking, 2010.

Guarneri, Mimi. *The Heart Speaks: A Cardiologist Reveals the Secret Language of Healing.* New York: Simon & Schuster, 2006.

Hay, Louise L. *You Can Heal Your Life.* Farmingdale, NY: Coleman, 1984.

Hendricks, Gay. *The Big Leap.* New York: HarperOne, 2009.

Hicks, Esther, and Jerry Hicks. *Ask and It Is Given: Learning to Manifest Your Desires.* Carlsbad, CA: Hay House, 2004.

Holick, Michael F. *The Vitamin D Solution: A 3-Step Strategy to Cure Our Most Common Health Problem.* New York: Hudson Street Press, 2010.

Holick, Michael. "Vitamin D Deficiency." *New England Journal of Medicine* 357(2007); 266-81. Print.

Holmes, Ernest. *The Science of Mind.* New York: Tarcher, 1998.

Kabat-Zinn, Jon. *Wherever You Go, There You Are.* New York: Hyperion, 2005.

—. *Full Catastrophe Living: Using the Wisdom of Your Body and Mind to Face Stress, Pain, and Illness.* New York: Delacorte Press, 1990.

Kasl, Charlotte Davis. *Finding Joy: 101 Ways to Free Your Spirit.* New York: HarperCollins, 1994.

Kataria, Madan. *Laugh for No Reason.* Mumbai: Madhuri, 1999.

Katie, Byron. *Loving What Is: Four Questions That Can Change Your Life.* New York: Harmony Books, 2002.

Kern, Deborah. *Everyday Wellness for Women.* Moulton, AL: Slaton Press, 1999.

Kristof, Nicholas D., and Sheryl WuDunn. *Half the Sky: Turning Oppression into Opportunity for Women Worldwide.* New York: Alfred A. Knopp, 2009.

Kübler-Ross, Elisabeth. *On Death and Dying.* New York: Maxwell Macmillan, 1993.

Lipton, Bruce. *The Biology of Belief: Unleashing the Power of Consciousness, Matter and Miracles.* Carlsbad, CA: Hay House, 2008.

Lipton, Bruce, and Steve Bhaerman. *Spontaneous Evolution: Our Positive Future (and a Way to Get There From Here).* Carlsbad, CA: Hay House, 2009.

MacWilliam, Lyle. *NutriSearch Comparative Guide to Nutritional Supplements.* Vernon, BC: Northern Dimensions, 2007.

Morrissey, Mary Manin. *No Less Than Greatness: Finding Perfect Love in Imperfect Relationships.* New York: Bantam Books, 2001.

Murray, Michelle W. "Laughter is the 'Best Medicine' for Your Heart." *Feature Stories.* University of Maryland Medical Center, 7 March 2005. Web. 21 Apr. 2007.

Myss, Caroline. *Anatomy of the Spirit.* New York: Three Rivers Press, 1996.

Northrup, Christiane. *Women's Bodies, Women's Wisdom.* New York: Bantam Books, 2010.

Orman, Suze. *The Courage to Be Rich: Creating a Life of Material and Spiritual Abundance.* New York: Riverhead Books, 1999.

Ornish, Dean. *Love & Survival: The Scientific Basis for the Healing Power of Intimacy.* New York: HarperCollins, 1998.

Pert, Candace. *Molecules of Emotion: The Science Behind Mind-Body Medicine.* New York: Scribner, 1997.

Roman, Sanaya, and Duane Packer. *Creating Money.* Tiburon, CA: H.J. Kramer Inc., 1988.

Rosas, Debbie, and Carlos Rosas. *The Nia Technique: The High-Powered Energizing Workout that Gives You a New Body and a New Life.* New York: Broadway Books, 2004.

Rosenberg, Marshall. *Nonviolent Communication: A Language of Life.* Encinitas, CA: PuddleDancer Press, 2003.

Ruiz, Don Miguel. *The Four Agreements.* San Rafael, CA: Amber-Allen, 1997.

Siegel, Bernie S. *Love, Medicine and Miracles: Lessons Learned about Self-Healing from a Surgeon's Experience with Exceptional Patients.* New York: Quill, 1990.

Strand, Ray D. *Healthy for Life.* Rapid City, SD: Real Life Press, 2005.

Stubbs, Kenneth Ray. *Sacred Orgasms.* Larkspur, CA: Secret Garden, 1993.

Taylor, Jill Bolte. *My Stroke of Insight: A Brain Scientist's Personal Journey.* New York: Viking Adult, 2007.

Tolle, Eckhart. *The Power of Now: A Guide to Spiritual Enlightenment.* Novato, CA: New World Library, 1999.

Walsch, Neale Donald. *The Little Soul and the Sun: A Children's Parable Adapted from Conversations with God.* Charlottesville, VA: Hampton Roads, 1998.

Weil, Andrew. *Spontaneous Healing: How to Discover and Enhance Your Body's Natural Ability to Maintain and Heal Itself.* New York: Ballantine, 1995.

Williamson, Marianne. *Enchanted Love: The Mystical Power of Intimate Relationships.* New York: Simon & Schuster, 1999.

Wolfe, Karen, and Deborah Kern. *Create the Body Your Soul Desires: The Friendship Solution to Weight, Energy and Sexuality.* Mission Viejo, CA: Healing Quest, 2003.

Reflection Pages

Reflection Pages

Reflection Pages

Reflection Pages

Reflection Pages

Reflection Pages

Reflection Pages

Reflection Pages

Reflection Pages

Reflection Pages

About the Author

SUSAN TATE is also the author of *Into the Mouths of Babes: A Natural Foods Nutrition and Feeding Guide for Infants and Toddlers*, *AIDS & HIV Education: Effective Teaching Strategies*, and *Working Together to Prevent Sexual Assault*. She is the director of Washington Wellness Associates and specializes in wellness consulting and the delivery of health education programs from an empowering, compassionate perspective. A respected health educator for over forty years, Susan served as the director of health promotion and assistant professor in the School of Medicine at the University of Virginia for many years. She is a black belt Nia instructor and delights in being a dancing grandmother.

Her passion for her work is evident in her life's intent—to inspire individual, community, and global wellness. Susan has two grown children and lives in Edmonds, Washington.

www.wawellness.com